We Beat the Beast

A Kidney Cancer Survivor's Story of Hope and Faith

By
Charles Piotrowski

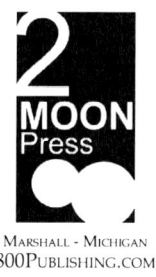

MARSHALL - MICHIGAN
800PUBLISHING.COM

We Beat the Beast: A Kidney Cancer Survivor's Story of Hope and Faith

Copyright © 2012 by Charles Piotrowski

Layout by Kait Lamphere

Author photo courtesy of author

The opinions expressed in this manuscript are solely the opinions of the author and do not represent the opinions or thoughts of the publisher. The author represents and warrants that s/he either owns or has the legal right to publish all material in this book.

ISBN-13: 978-1-938110-31-3

First published in 2012

10 9 8 7 6 5 4 3 2 1

Published by   2 MOON PRESS
123 W. Michigan Ave, Marshall, Michigan 49068
www.800publishing.com

All Rights Reserved. This book may not be reproduced, transmitted, or stored in whole or in part by any means, including graphic, electronic, or mechanical without the express written consent of the publisher except in the case of brief quotations embodied in critical articles and reviews.

PRINTED IN THE UNITED STATES OF AMERICA

This book is being dedicated to my wife Jeannie.
I could not have beaten cancer without her at my side.
Throughout this ordeal she walked with me.

I affectionately referred to her as "The Warden;"
she watched my every move.

She is my best friend. She is my caregiver. She is my personal chef. She is my prayer partner. She is my social secretary. The list goes on and on. She does it all, always, always, always!

In Mitch Albom's play <u>Ernie</u>, there is an exchange between Ernie and his wife LuLu and the tremendous love they shared. They were married for 68 years. Ernie was asked how long their honeymoon was and he said, "I'll let you know when it's over." Kind of like my love with Jeannie!

Thank you Jeannie, I LOVE YOU!!

Prologue

Who is the "We" referred to in the title of this book? It is everyone who has touched my life. I am not strong enough to have beaten this beast alone. The doctors certainly are smart enough. But beating cancer is more than having the medical knowledge. Prayer is an important part of this process, but we do need the doctors.

And then there is the social aspect. Having my family and friends to pick me up when I was down was essential. And having those same people with me in times of joy was equally important. Perhaps I could have named this book, "You Beat the Beast!" That doesn't seem appropriate because it is a delicate balance among a lot of "yous." And I have beaten cancer four times.

In 2004 I had a tumor in my duodenum that was <u>benign</u>. In February of 2011, I was diagnosed with kidney cancer, which was successfully removed through surgery. And in April 2011, a "suspicious spot" on my lower spine was biopsied – to find out that it was <u>not cancer</u>. And in June, three small growths were found on my lungs. After testing, those growths were found to be irrelevant. They do bear observation, but <u>at this time they are not cancer</u>!!

So – **We** have Beaten the Beast four times, surrounded by the grace of God!! *We* can do it; *we* can do anything! WOO-HOO! It is so exciting. This book is about the support all of you have provided. I have never felt more surrounded by love than I have through these four incidents, especially the three in 2011. My purpose in writing this book is the hope that maybe one other person will receive help from reading my story. Somebody loved me through this and I am going to "Pay it Forward" and love somebody else through this as well. All I hope for is one, but the more the merrier.

One concern I have with the word WE is that many of the WE will be mentioned in these pages. The WE includes people who have called, emailed, texted, sent a card, Facebooked, used an entry on Caring Bridge, and/or who have stopped in to pay a visit. Some of these visits are documented through the means in which the visit occurred. Other visits, although greatly appreciated, go unrecorded. As I sit down to write this book, I thank all of the WE. There is always a danger of unintentionally omitting a person's name. So I start now by offering an apology to anyone who I walked with, but their name does not appear in this book. Each person who walked with me knows how important their role is/was. And I know I have been challenged by all of you to be more present to walking with others who need loving, prayerful support throughout the rest of my life. I hope that you, too, will be up to that challenge. It just involves two key elements – both of which we have lots of: Love and Time!

One of my Burger King customers has an important rule in his life. He does everything "All for the Glory of God!" He learned years ago that being another member of the rat race is not enough. He wants to make a difference. He is a self-employed contractor. On his truck he has painted "All for the Glory of God!" The same inscription is also found on all of his business cards--kind of a neat theme to embody. Try it on for size.

God is Good, All the Time! All the Time, God is Good!!

Chapter 1
Who Am I and Where Am I Going?

... Humble Beginnings

If you are lucky enough to own a copy of the October 25, 1951, *Chicago Daily News* (as I am – thanks to a 55th birthday present from TR), you can skim the paper for all kinds of information as to what was going on in the world that day. Amazingly, the paper itself only cost five cents for home delivery, as opposed to the $1.00 one pays in 2011. The headline for that magnificent day read that the naval fleet was ready to use the Atomic bomb in the Mediterranean Sea if it were deemed necessary (what does necessary mean?).

It was warm on that October day in 1951, 63 degrees at twelve noon. There was a picture in the first section with the following caption, "Start work with a prayer!" (How times have changed). The three headline movies of that day only cost 19 cents and included Mickey Rooney in <u>The Strip</u>, Jane Wyman in <u>The Blue Veil</u>, and Burt Lancaster in <u>Jim Thorpe, All American</u>. The Dow Jones Stock average on that cheery Thursday was a whopping 232. In football, the Wisconsin Badgers were leading the Big Ten. The paper was filled with articles about the big fight, Rocky Marciano vs. Joe Louis. (Marciano did overpower Detroit's Joe Louis two days later). There was speculation as to whether or not Joe DiMaggio would actually retire. He had announced his retirement on September 30, but many thought he would reconsider (he didn't). Richard McGraw was the 9th jockey killed in 1951. A person could rent an apartment for $35.00 a month and buy a five room brick house with a garage for $17,000. A used 1950 Pontiac Sedan, with low mileage, was available for $1,695.

Prices for food and clothing at the time really emphasize what inflation has done since. A pair of "Father and Son" shoes was $6.95. A

Hathaway shirt was $5.95 and the silk tie to go with it was on sale for $2.35. Bargains at the supermarket included two bars of Lux soap for 23 cents. A large bottle of Ketchup was only 19 cents. A head of lettuce, 13 cents. Those with a sweet tooth could buy three boxes of Cracker Jack for 25 cents, and the toy was real. If you were into chewing gum, three packs of Wrigley's cost ten cents. A pound of bacon was 49 cents, while a pound of coffee was a staggering 77 cents. And we all love our pets (well maybe not I), so a proud dog owner could buy a one pound can of dog food for nine cents.

This was the world into which I was born on October 25, 1951. It was a bright world and it was filled with promises for me and my generation; Baby Boomers we were to be nicknamed.

... My Heritage

I was the first born son of Hank and Rita Piotrowski. My parents were born in 1919 and 1925, respectively. They both struggled through the years of the Depression. They certainly knew the true value of the dollar better than most Baby Boomers. To know me is to know my family. Family is a theme that is sooo important to me. Whether it is my family of origin, my extended family, my work family, my school family, my neighborhood family – whatever the case, I am proud to be a member of THAT family and will do my best to be a family member to the fullest.

In the case of my parents, their number one priority was family. Their whole life centered on making things better for their family. They were willing to sacrifice everything for their kids. It is a trait for which I will be eternally grateful. It is a trait which I try to live today. It is a trait that I hope to pass on to my children. Birthday celebrations and special events were celebrated at our home in St. Clair Shores with family (no surprise there) and a few close friends, who were really extended family. It was a simple life, but so profound. As with so many married couples of that era, my parents rarely said the words, "I Love You" out loud, but their actions expressed that sentiment several times each day.

Hank Piotrowski was a hard-working, fun-loving man. He was definitely the traditional "head of the house." He ruled the roost. Many times we had to honor his wishes because, "I said so", even though there appeared to be no logical reason. Hank was a butcher at Kroger, owned his own party store with my mom, and then worked some factory jobs prior to his retirement. He loved collecting stamps and coins; there was no money to do that when he was a kid. He loved dabbling in the stock market, always hoping to make that killing. He had a passion for writing and drawing. He used three-by-five cards to exercise that skill and sent my sister and me a daily message when we worked at camp or were at college – that was one of the many ways he said, "I Love You".

He had some "Hankisms," things that he said *ad nauseum.* The first demonstrates that he was a man filled with ethics: "It's not whether you win or lose, it's how you play the game." And he practiced what he preached. The second "Hankism" demonstrated how important it was for him to work hard: "You don't get nothing for nothing." Hank was definitely a Piotrowski – patience was not one of his attributes, a claim that I can confirm to this day. I can remember wetting my pants as a kid when he played chicken with another black Ford sedan on I-94, weaving in and out of traffic, because the other driver cut him off during a lane change. The whole time we was laying on the horn and calling the other driver a "Farmer" (he died before he could explain that term of endearment to me).

The last "Hankism" I want to share centers around my youngest son, Matthew. By the time Matt was born, Hank was in the last three years of his life. He really could focus on Matt and enjoy him. Hank did not have many other things to occupy his time. I am not sure what Hank saw in Matt, but every time he saw Matt he uttered, "He's gonna be something else." Although he used that term with Matt, it is a term which he could use with any of his eight grandchildren. In many ways the love of his life was his grandkids. Whether he was cheering on Mikey at a hockey game (hollering, "Hustle") or watching Joe in a Gabriel Richard stage play (which Hank did just six days before he died) – he was one proud grandpa. In reality, Hank Piotrowski was "something else!"

Behind every great man is a great woman; Rita "Reet" Piotrowski fits that bill. She started each day with a cup of Sanka and ended it watching Johnny Carson on a TV (no remote control) in the front room. The Depression was especially hard on my mom. Her mother would buy a steak for dinner. Her dad got to eat the steak (he was the one who worked) and everyone else got to eat a soup made from the steak juices. Grandpa Costello died when mom was 12 and she left school to help provide money for the family of five kids by scooping ice cream at Schweitzer's in Detroit. Without an eighth grade education, my mom was one of the smartest women I knew. She was always there to back my dad. She complemented him, but also lost her own identity. She was subservient for sure. She didn't even drive a car until she was in her 50s. Shortly thereafter she went out to buy her own first car. Hank gave her two instructions; make no mistake they were definitely instructions/orders. The car had to be a Ford and could be any color but white. I can still see the look on Hank's face when "Reet" pulled up in a White Pontiac Grand Prix. Fortunately, Hank learned to enjoy that white sports car.

Many of my memories of "Reet" center around the Handee Food Centre, located at 805 Goddard in Wyandotte. It was her life and almost cost her that precious life. She was up at 5 a.m. daily cooking and cleaning before opening the store. Then at 4 p.m. daily (she didn't drive back then) she walked that half mile to our home, whatever the weather was, to help us with our homework and prepare a tasty dinner. I miss her homemade "Reet" rolls and her tasty homemade desserts (store-bought was not an option). Treats at the store were also not an option – that would cut into the profit. She loved her little eight ounce bottles of Coke. She always had one on the counter. As kids we would sneak up to "steal a swig." Secretly, we hoped to get caught because my mom would not ever drink out of a bottle that somebody else's lips had touched – so the Coke became ours! That trick worked for years. I believe it was her way of giving us a pop without giving us a pop. But, my mom was a germ-freak; she never gave us a kiss on the lips. I always wondered what kind of germs she thought she would get from her own kids.

A major change in the life of my folks happened on a fall day in

1971. Mom was alone in the store while dad was buying supplies. An alleged customer came in and ordered a pack of cigarettes. When my mom turned her back on the customer, the drug-crazed freak hit her over the head with a hammer. It nearly killed her and did distort her vision for the rest of her life. Jim (the Hostess cupcake guy) walked in as this was transpiring – he too got to experience that damn hammer. It did change my parents' lives. There was no more joy at Handee Food Centre and the store was for sale the next day.

Hank went home to the Lord in 1997. He was sitting in his favorite easy chair, with a toothpick behind his ear. He was listening to J.P. McCarthy on WJR and had just finished discussing stocks with his best friend, Stan Sarnacki. Mom had made his lunch and called him to eat. He did not respond. She went into the front room and discovered him dead of an apparent heart attack. Being an aficionado of sweets, it was appropriate to serve his favorite rice pudding at the funeral lunch.

Rita died in 2004. She had been in failing health, but was so independent. She would sit outside pulling weeds and scoot along on her butt, because she was so proud of that home on 10th Street. Her laundry became my responsibility. She asked me if I minded and I said that it was fine, but I did admit to her that it was a little disconcerting washing her undies. A few days later I noticed there were no undies to wash. I figured she was washing them in the sink. I apologized for mentioning it to her and told her to throw her undies in with the dirty laundry. She smiled and said that since it bothered me she would no longer wear any underwear – and she never did. Mom was so angry with me when she found it necessary to place her in the nursing home next to Seaway Hospital. She wanted to go back to 10th Street. The doc insisted on inserting a feeding tube, as she was not eating. I knew my mom would resist that so I told the doc no. He said, "We'll just see." We approached my mom together and he expressed his desire. She looked at me and said, "He knows better than that – no feeding tube." I just smiled and said to myself, "I told you so."

When it was obvious her time was limited, Ron Victor came and anointed her and she went to her beloved home on 10th Street for her last six days. The care she received from her Guardian Angel, Nadine, was awesome. We gathered around mom's bed the night before she died, not even knowing if she knew we were there. My friend and classmate (Ron Victor) celebrated the funeral of both my parents – what a personal touch. And in my mom's case, Fr. Ed Prus was the concelebrant. Following the tradition of my dad, her funeral luncheon was also topped off with a sweet – a banana split - which was the last food of any sustenance she ate before her death.

I am so proud of both of my parents that they each donated their bodies for research purposes to the U of M. At a U of M Memorial service six months later, a doctor spoke and thanked the donor families who were present for the unselfish donation of the bodies of their loved ones. There wasn't a dry eye in the house.

The man I am today can certainly be linked to my parents. They challenged each of their children to be the best that we could be. And their challenge was one that was not verbalized, rather it was demonstrated by the way they lived their lives. What an awesome example.

... *Grade School Years*

I was educated at St. Lucy's in St. Clair Shores and Mt. Carmel in Wyandotte. I was smart enough, but not really a stand-out. My sister (Patsy – born in November of 1952) and my brother (TR – born In February of 1954) were one and three years behind me. My sister and I fought like all brothers and sisters. As my parents were often at the "store", my sister had an ally in her friend across the street. Helen Sarnacki was Patsy's guardian angel. I can still remember pushing Patsy in the snow for probably no reason. I walked in the door and Helen was already on the phone, threatening me. I do remember several times of discipline, when I received the brunt of the discipline because I was the oldest and it was my responsibility to set a better example. I often wanted to switch birth order with either of my siblings.

My dad's mom died when I was in the third grade. His boss gave him two box seats to a Tiger game at Briggs Stadium; a different expression of sympathy It was my first game. I don't remember who won, but I was there with my dad. This started a life-long devotion of the Tigers. A few years later the entire family went to a game when my Uncle John and his family were visiting from California. It was the only game my mom ever attended. There was a long foul ball hit in the area where we were seated. My dad moved with lightning speed, something I was not accustomed to seeing. He followed the flight of the ball and rolled around on the floor fighting a teenager for the ball. Hank got the ball and promptly gave it to my cousin Dick; I was ticked.

In the seventh grade I thought of eventually entering the seminary. The nuns loved it. I went from a B-C student to an all A student overnight. Needing to be prepared for the seminary, I began to practice the Mass. As many of my friends did, I celebrated Mass in the basement at a work bench which my dad had made (I still have that work bench/altar in my garage). I used Ritz crackers and grape juice and wore my bath robe for a chasuble. TR was kind enough (I must have bribed him) to be the congregation. And what did I preach about?? The same things that I heard priests preach about (and still do today) - the need for the parishioners to do a better job with their contributions--seems to be a common theme.

... *High School Years*

I entered high school at Sacred Heart Seminary (Cardinal Mooney Latin School) in September of 1965. My grades were in the B-C range. Those grade school Felician nuns spoiled me into believing I was an all "A" student. Imagine my shock when I got a "D" in religion of all subjects; it was quite a shock. It was during this time that I met one of the "Rocks" in my life. Fr. Ed Prus taught me freshman English and was also the Spiritual Director. Calling him a "Rock" might be an understatement. He once defined prayer as: "wasting time with Jesus." What a simple yet profound definition. And Fr. Prus not only talked the talk, but he walked the walk. Forty five years later, I am proud and honored to call Fr. Prus my friend. Another memory of Fr. Prus is the weekly essays that he demanded we write. What a chore that was; for me it was impossible. We had to present a draft by Wednesday and then the final essay on Friday. I never got above a "C". Steve "Eli"

Whitney always won the coveted Oleo Lae testiae trophy, for the best written paragraph. I never came close. But who knows, the seed for this book could have been born in those essays.

Relationships are so important. In my freshman year I met Ron Victor, Jay Yule, Mike Morris, Mike Meyers, and Rick Klapchar – they are the epitome of a fraternity. All of these men and their families are still so close to me. We are there for each other in good times and in bad. We always have a group picture taken when together at one of our kids' weddings for "the good times." I am so proud and fortunate to be surrounded by such fine people. We are really all one large extended family.

It was during these my High School years that I acted on a suggestion of the school guidance counselor, Fr. Bill Doran. He felt that I would mature faster and learn how to interact better if I joined a staff at a summer camp. (Geez, was I an introvert back then?) There were two choices – Camp Sancta Maria in Gaylord (where the "rich kids" went) or Camp Ozanam in Port Sanilac, sponsored by the Society of St. Vincent de Paul (SVdP). Campers were given a two week **free** camping experience. As you will see as my life story unfolds, I am so happy that I chose Camp Ozanam. I ended up working 14 summers at Ozanam, and then another 17 years for the stores operation of SVdP. The Camp Ozanam motto is one I will never forget, "Accept, Share, and Develop." They are three principles I try to embody even today.

I truly received a wonderful life foundation during those years. Living in the center of the city, I experienced life within a Black community during this time. I was there during the assassinations of Dr. Martin Luther King Jr., and Robert F. Kennedy, and lived with the reaction of the community. I even shook hands earlier with RFK as his motorcade swung by Sacred Heart Seminary during one of his campaign tours. During the '67 riots somebody painted the face of statue of the Sacred Heart black. It caused a ruckus and an anonymous person repainted the face white. The rector, Msgr. Canfield, had the face repainted black and let it be known that it was to remain that way. And to this day in 2011 it is still black. God is not bounded by color or gender.

1968 saw the Detroit Tigers beat the St. Louis Cardinals in the

World Series. A number of us were at the game when the Tigers clinched the pennant. I ran on the field, excited as the rest. I had one of the old tan seat covers and wanted to scoop up some of the dirt by 1st base and present it to Ron Victor, as a souvenir from the spot which Ron's hero (Norm Cash) inhabited. I was stopped by one of Detroit's "finest" and threatened with jail, if I didn't drop it immediately. Needless to say, I dropped it and, my record is clean.

I was so thrilled in June of 1969 to receive my High school diploma from Fr. Art Schaffran and Msgr. Canfield; and somehow that faculty recommended that I be allowed to move on to Sacred Heart Seminary College and continue on my journey to priesthood. And the five cronies I mentioned earlier (along with some other fine men) were continuing on with me.

One final reflection on my high school years centers on music. At the end of our junior year we had to take a final exam for Christian Living. After the normal annoying multiple guess questions (oh how I hated those), we were asked to analyze the lyrics to a then-popular Judy Collins song, <u>Both Sides Now.</u> I did it then and I do it now; it is quite an impactful song. Two other songs from our senior year were <u>The</u> <u>Impossible Dream</u> and <u>Feelin' Groovy (59th Street Bridge Street</u>). Those songs entered my life over forty years ago and still impact me today – much more than thousands of songs I have learned since then. Do yourself a favor and go online to read those lyrics. *(Besides it is easier than my getting permission to reprint those lyrics and I also do not have to type them).*

... College Years

The four years of college went fairly smoothly. Sad to admit now, I was very lazy as far as being a student. (Thank God my kids did not follow my example!) My grades were satisfactory. Had I put forth the effort in my academics that I did in other areas, I would have excelled scholastically, but that was not me.

I became influenced by two more of my "Rocks" during my college career. The next one was Mr. Jerry Brown. He was the first

African American employee at Sacred Heart Seminary (SHS). He ended up employed there for a total of 50 years, quite an accomplishment in any work environment. He was initially hired as a dishwasher, moved up to run the entire kitchen, and was plant manager at the time of his retirement. I loved the stories that man could tell, simple yet profound. Most mornings at 6:30 a.m. I began my day in his office in the basement of St. Joe's Hall. I believe I received a substantial education from Professor Brown. His field of expertise was in educating me about the black society, and he educated me about helping the downtrodden. Together, he and I founded the seminary soup kitchen which was housed in the old Powerhouse. Not only did we feed the downtrodden daily, but we were also there for conversation and a place to lift their spirits, and many wintery days we provided necessary shelter. Brilliant men and women helped me to encounter the academics, but Professor Brown taught me about life. He was presented an award by the Alumni Association of the Seminary. I was excited to attend his ceremony. Imagine my shock when I asked him before the ceremony what he was going to speak about. He looked at me with that toothy grin of his and said, "P, I am not speaking tonight – I am going to have you give my speech." What an honor it was to speak about this "Doctor of Life."

It was also during my college years that I met another "Rock" in my life – Sr. Mary Finn. I have admired Sister Mary for over forty years. She influenced my life in two ways. She taught me the simplicity of prayer–you don't have to plan for it, just do it. Even now I can hear her say, "It's kind of a mystery." Sr. Mary was also involved in the local community and at SHS she was assigned as faculty moderator of the Christian Apostolate. I was fortunate enough to be the student representative, working closely with her to provide ministerial opportunities for all students, in addition to their classroom education. Our seminary education was truly three-fold: Prayer, ministry, and classroom – all three were important in the enrichment of us all. Sr. Mary takes advantage of every opportunity. Still today as she is leaving a conversation she gives you a warm hug, and, while she hugs you, she traces the sign of the cross on your back. Go in peace with the Lord! She truly inspires me - I am enthralled whenever I have the opportunity to speak with her. Today we shared notes on cancer. Twenty three years ago, she was diagnosed with colon cancer and had her surgery on Jeannie's birthday 23 years ago. Sr. Mary being the epitome of spirituality would chose the above title for her book, "Befriend My Cancer." She explains that she spoke these words to cancer as she dealt with its reality, "I will not fight you because you will win. You are living in my body, my house." What an attitude. I should have spoken with Sr. Mary as I was dealing with my cancer. Instead of struggling to beat the beast, I would have made more of an effort to befriend my cancer. That is why Sr. Mary is one of my "rocks" and not vice versa.

On December 8, 1972, I reached the decision that priesthood was not my goal. In that I only had one more semester left to receive my B.A. in History, I decided to complete my education at SHS. It was a proud day in April of 1973 when I received my College Diploma from John Cardinal Dearden. What an awesome moment it was to walk across the auditorium stage in my tennis shoes and receive that glorious piece of parchment.

... Bachelor Years

So who am I and where am I going? I have just left eight years in the seminary and had no clue in which direction my life was heading. My first step was the same step I took every summer – I headed to Camp Ozanam. How I loved that experience. And I know that I learned more from those campers than I was ever able to give them.

The summer ended and I was lost. It was the first time in my life I felt empty and lonely. Most of my friends had moved on to St. John's Seminary. The others who had left had definite career paths. I had nothing. I moped and felt sorry for myself. My parents would not allow it – they demanded that I go out and find a JOB. What was a man with a BA in History qualified to do? I scanned the want ads and found the perfect fit. I went to Professional Bartender's School. Many of my friends kidded me that I was qualified to hear confessions from behind the bar. I worked in two different establishments. My first stop was a red-neck saloon in Flat Rock. Then I graduated to an upscale tavern in Detroit, Pat O'Grady's. A couple years earlier I wore tennis shoes to graduation and now I was wearing a white shirt and tie to work every day. I will always be grateful to Pat and Karla for giving me the opportunity for my first real job. During those years I learned a lot about serving others. Eventually I moved into management. I learned about the necessary balance between taking care of customers and taking care of employees.

    The constant in my life continued to be Camp Ozanam. No matter where I was employed, the management was always gracious enough to allow me to have the summers off to be on the shores of Lake Huron. In the late 70s my dad was unemployed and we needed a cook at Camp, so Hank took the job. In addition to cooking, he loved umping baseball games, playing the role of Hanko the Clown, and leading the Indian pageantry as Chief Muckleshoot. It was a thrill to work in that environment with my dad. To be honest, my dad was a bit of a racist. As I mentioned earlier, patience was not a Piotrowski trait. He could get very frustrated and use some racial slurs that he would later regret. By the end of his camp experience, Hank saw the beauty of people of all races and was proud of it. I was proud to be part of that growth process.

    During the first week of camp in the summer of 1978, the Kitchen Manager at Camp Stapleton (the sister camp to Ozanam) needed help repairing the camp dishwasher. Being as un-mechanical as they come, I did a great job faking it. I don't know if they ever had clean dishes at Camp Stapleton, but I met the true "Love of my Life," the phenomenal Jeannie Byron. As the summer wore along, we made lots of excuses to be together. Oh my gosh, I was falling in love. The day after Thanksgiving in 1978, sitting on two bar stools in Pat O'Grady's we agreed to get married. Neither one of us proposed, it was just a given–the next logical step. An August 1979 wedding was planned.

    Due to a change of leadership at O'Grady's, it was time for this man with a BA in history and five years of bartending experience to find other work. Not an overwhelming resume, but I found work rather easily. In fact, I was hired sitting on a different bar stool at Pat O'Grady's. The St. Vincent de Paul Society ran a Stores Operation. The main purpose of that operation was to provide furniture, appliances, and clothing to the poor. Their secondary purpose was to provide funding for that camp operation that was such an important part of my life. It seemed like a perfect fit–so my professional life took another turn. I was able to make great use of the things taught to me by the three "rocks" of my life, Fr. Prus, Jerry Brown, and Sr. Mary Finn. It was the hardest physical work of my life. The store was virtually bankrupt when I joined their team. I am proud to say that, as a team, we made a difference. By the time my tenure there ended 17 years later, we were annually distributing over $1,000,000 of goods to the needy and providing hundreds of thousands of dollars to the Camping operation annually.

... Married Life

The summer of 1979 was the last summer in my tenure at Camp Ozanam. It was increasingly special because we were planning our wedding. And planning our wedding two hours away from our families was hard and easy; hard because of logistics, easy because we did it all alone without any interference, sorry mom (but not really).

In mid-June 1979, we were thrown a curve ball. My dear friend and co-worker from Pat O'Grady's, Gary Victor, committed suicide. To this day, it remains the single most devastating instance in my life. I can remember that phone call like it was yesterday. Logically I know that I did all that I could to help. I will always wonder IF I could have done something else. Life is too valuable to give up that easily. It is not a bad thing to ask for professional help, as will be discussed later.

Preparing for our wedding and living life within the Byron/Loeffler family introduced me to the next "Rock" in my life – Uncle (Fr.) Earl. What a gem he was. Uncle Earl was a passionate educator and a wonderful pastor. And, upon retirement, his favorite ministry was to the prisoners at Milan prison. Whichever ministry Uncle Earl was involved in, he gave 100%. What I learned the most from him was to roll with the punches. He was most progressive in his thinking. He knew how to write letters and to diplomatically challenge authority.

He saw an important role for lay people and women in the leadership of the church and in the daily ministry of the church. He was a man ahead of his time. And any of us who were lucky enough to be around him were enriched by his presence. I enjoyed being in his presence at family gatherings and compared it to Jesus preaching to people on the hillside. He had "High Hopes." Jeannie and I were lucky to invite him and Ron Victor to concelebrate our wedding.

What an awesome celebration August 24, 1979 was. Three hundred fifty people converged on St. Clement Church and then the Shores Hall. The night is a blur – to have all of our loved ones in the same building was so special. I could feel the love!! We wrote our own vows – unfortunately we did not save a copy. The theme of the vows was "unconditional love." And thirty-two years later that unconditional love is stronger than ever.

One of the more embarrassing moments of our lives came three days later on August 27. We received a call from "Hans", the owner of the Shores Hall. He was angry and upset. The check that we used to pay for our wedding reception had bounced. I told him that was impossible–he was not buying my story. Realize the year was 1979; electronic transfers of money and computer usage were not prevalent. The check was drawn on the Bank of Croswell. The money did not go from Croswell to St. Clair Shores as quickly as we anticipated, hence the bounced check. The funds finally cleared the bank and all lived happily ever after, especially Hans.

We chose to honeymoon over New Year's Eve in Las Vegas. My brother TR and his wife (Barb) went with us. It was a four day party. It's a little different to share your honeymoon with your brother, but we have a strong relationship. And on New Year's Eve we listened to an amazing performance by Sister Sledge. And their number one hit at the time was, "We Are Family." That is what this book is all about; the beauty of family, both the blood relatives and the extended family.

... Kids

Joseph Charles (2-10-82) was our first born. He was followed months later by his sister Ellen Byron (6-8-83). Jeannie and I were in training to be parents (is that a course that you ever complete?). What a joyful addition they were to our lives. I was asked what quality I felt was most important to instill in our children. Without hesitating I responded, "A sense of humor." Being an academician, I am not sure that Jeannie agreed with me. Jeannie worked on school work and I handled social skills. And as I am writing this almost 30 years later, I think we did fairly well. Sure we made mistakes, but we worked together and kept our **family** intact. Due to a situation at Gabriel Richard, Jeannie was called in to work. What to do with Joey? Hank Pio to the rescue. Hank never did much in the raising of his own children and now here he was changing Joey's diaper. And he sang all of those country songs daily. And it is interesting that all three of my kids have affection for country music, which will never be in my Top Ten.

Rita had a special relationship with Ellen, especially on half days of school. Grandma would take her to McDonald's (there wasn't a convenient Burger King nearby) and grandma would have a small fry and a coffee, while Ellen ate her kid's meal. Hank and Rita were involved in their grandkids' lives. Ellen was quite the opposite of Joe. Joe slept through the night his first night home. Ellen didn't stop crying for the first two years; the "Soprano of Netherwood," is what she was christened by our nearest neighbors. They were so different, but so similar. We love them so much!

... *October, 1984*

I am addicted to the Tigers. Sparky Anderson led the '84 Tigers on quite a ride. They started the season with a 35-5 run and then just had to maintain from there. What I would have given to go to the World Series against the dreaded San Diego Padres. My mother-in-law sent in a ticket request and her entry was pulled out of the hat. She had four seats and 16 people who wanted to use them. The first two went to the parents, of course. So now there were two seats and fourteen takers. A lottery was held. Unbelievably, Jeannie's name and mine were the first two names pulled. We sat in the upper deck in left field. I still remember Kirk Gibson's home run and Larry Herndon's catch to end the game. We partied with the rest of the celebrating fans. Imagine our surprise when we read the paper the next day and learned of the rioting that was caused by that victory. In a short time frame, Detroit was celebrating and embarrassed.

... Back to the Family

Five years later we were thrilled when Jeannie became pregnant again. We were surprised that it took so long, but we figured God was in charge. Jeannie went for a routine checkup and we were stunned to learn that there was no heartbeat. Our third child had stopped living before being born. Many times over the years I have wondered WHY. And we will never know the answer. We have our faith to rely on and we did, even though it hurt so much.

In the summer of 1993, Jeannie didn't feel well. Her symptoms lead us both to wonder if she could be pregnant. It could not be possible, Jeannie was 40 and we had not had a child in twelve years. Due to the miscarriage, we wanted to keep it a secret until we were absolutely certain. We bought half a dozen pregnancy tests from the drug store. They all confirmed our suspicions. What a joy!! Now, to tell Joe and Ellen. We thought we were being cautious, but they had figured it out with little clues we had given including the before-mentioned EPT kits from CVS. The pregnancy went off without a hitch and Matthew Thomas was born on May 2, 1994. His name means "gift from the Lord", and he truly was. Due to the gap in our children's ages, Matt was really raised by four adults–poor kid. Of course he was also spoiled by four adults. And there was always Grandpa Hank who would look at Matt and continually say, "He is gonna' be something else". In many ways, by the time Matt came around, we learned kids don't break. I feel we were much more relaxed. When we dropped a pacifier, we didn't rush to boil water we just wiped it on our pants and shoved it in Matt's mouth. Maybe that's why he has turned out the way he has. And as I write this, Matt has just completed his junior year at Gabriel Richard.

All the while we were raising these adorable kids, my work continued at St. Vincent de Paul. 1980 was the first summer in 14 years that I spent in the metropolitan area. It was so blasted hot, and Jeannie reminded me we no longer had the cool breezes of Lake Huron to cool us off at night. I enjoyed my work immensely at SVdP. And I was filled with pride as I saw the amount of goods given away (the value of donated gifts exceeded $1,000,000 per year) and the amount of surplus generated grow each year. It was a business and we formed a solid team to make that business grow. It was tragic in December of 1995 when a fire occurred which burned down the entire block that housed our headquarters. It was one of the sadder days of my life. But the Society did recover from those ashes and I was proud to be a part of that process.

... 1989

One of the most humbling events of my life came in 1989. Sacred Heart Seminary named me the lay alumnus of the year, giving me the Walter Romig Award. That award still hangs proudly today in my office. I have always attributed that award to my work at St. Vincent de Paul. A few pages ago, I commented that I was lazy as a student. That just added to the amazement of being the recipient of this award. It was special that many of my former professors were in attendance that night. There certainly were many other worthy candidates, but I sure was proud to win and still appreciate the recognition. Humbled again! The award was actually presented by Fr. Pat Halfpenny (a few years older than me) who will be mentioned later in the book.

... Professional Life after St. Vinnies

Unfortunately, the Society decided to change leadership and their new Executive Director had a vision with which I could not work. I had learned a lot about the business world and was ready to take that knowledge and branch out on my own. I spoke with "Brother T" and sought his input. We both agreed that it would be a wise idea to apply for my own Burger King franchise here in Michigan. The approval process was long and tedious. Once I was approved, I had to find the right site to build. Burger King strongly suggested some areas, which I deemed unbuildable for various reasons. Then Jeannie and I found a vacant piece of property in Whitmore Lake, thus a Burger King at 9774 E. M-36 was born. Construction was a nightmare as we discovered our "perfect" site was a former dump. We had to remove four hundred tires, the front end of a car, and six refrigerators, among other things. Through it all our business sprung up. October 1, 1996 was opening day. It was the culmination and fulfillment of my latest dream.

Business was very brisk and profitable. Then two major things changed the course of action. First, US 23 (the freeway adjacent to our restaurant) was closed for road work. As we depend on that freeway for our customer base, sales came to a screeching halt. Road construction completed, we were ready for a quick rebound, but that was not to be. America's economy got punched in the belly, and Michigan endured more punches than most states. People did not have money to spend on their Whoppers. Thankfully, I did not spend the profits from those early years frivolously. And thankfully TR and I were partners on the real estate portion of this enterprise.

... My Brother (The Original Rock)

Now seems like an appropriate time to digress and talk about Brother T – TR. When I was 14, I left home to go to the seminary. TR was only 12. We did not know each other. I was effectively gone for eight years, and during summer vacation I was at Camp Ozanam; another lost opportunity to bond. We were fortunate enough to serve as "best man" at each other's weddings. As we grew into adulthood, we began to form an alliance that is so strong today. His life ended up being consumed by Burger King and his 11 restaurants in Indiana. I went from Pat O'Grady's to St. Vincent de Paul. In 1995, when I realized that it was time for a change, TR was right there to help me realize the opportunity in Burger King. Hence the alliance of Pio Bros, Inc., became a reality. To this day we speak on the phone minimally once a day, but multiple calls are a more likely scenario. We laugh at how frequently we talk, and often times have a hard time remembering what we even talked about. I am blessed to have a brother as wonderful as TR. I defy anyone to find two brothers as close as we are.

... *Minor Health Concerns*

I have been overweight most of my adult life. I was always ready to start that next diet, which never brought about any change. In the early 90s I was diagnosed as a diabetic. My dad was also a diabetic, but he always had a plethora of candy on the shelves in his bedroom. My eating habits were not much better than his. The more sugar you ate, the more insulin you took – not the sharpest knife in the drawer; it was a course of action that worked. I learned how to play the game, and what a dangerous game it was. I also had a problem with kidney stones – ouch! Thinking about them makes me wince. I can plainly recall my last instance of kidney stones in early 2004. I drove myself to the emergency room at Wyandotte Hospital. The docs discovered I was also anemic. Being the wise man I was, I disagreed with their observation. Once they confirmed their diagnosis, despite my disagreement, they set about to discover the root of the anemia. AHA! They encountered a tumor in my duodenum and it had to come out. The surgery was performed at U of M on June 7, 2004. The last thing I did before entering the hospital was to stop at Gabriel Richard for a Mass and pray for Divine Guidance. The surgery was very successful. The duration of the surgery was predicted at 5 hours and it took 8 ½ - I was out of it, but my poor family struggled for the last three hours. The doctors were very reassuring all along that they felt the tumor was benign, but it was a tremendous relief to KNOW, following the surgery, that the tumor was definitely benign. This was the first time that "We Beat the Beast!" I endured a two week hospital stay and was sent home to convalesce. I am not a fast healer and the whole process took a good six months, but I was raring to go and most appreciative of the wonderful care at U of M. It was a good lesson of reality for me. I was not invincible. I was human and I needed time to rejoin the hustle and bustle of daily life. It was during that summer of 2004 that my mom's health rapidly declined and I was able to walk with her through her final days at the nursing home and on 10th Street. I was happy to be there for her. I really developed affection for the staff at the hospital and the nursing home. The work they do is a true ministry. And what awesome ministers they were to my mom.

... I Get By With a Little Help from My Friends

Time for a true confession here. Anxiety was getting the best of me. I could not relax. I could not sleep at night. I was a perpetual worry-wart. I was driving myself nuts (and probably most of the people around me). I needed help. Males never need help. Heads of families never need help. I needed help. I pursued help with my local pastor. He told me I was nuts. I agreed with him and told him again that I needed help. He still did not take me serious – but he referred me to a magnificent lady who would become the next "Rock" of my life. Sr. Betty Leon was my lifeline. Over the years she has become a lifeline to others in my family as well. She listens and she cares. Men do not like to admit their weaknesses, especially those that seem to be mental or emotional in their nature. I am so glad I was not afraid to ask for help, I know it saved my life. Guys, there is nothing wrong with having a therapist, counselor, life coach, or whatever name you chose to designate. Sr. Betty often talks about setting up boundaries and expectations. Duh – it's not that hard, but I complicate things. She challenged me to carry around a Stop sign, and not let that "stinkin' thinkin'" into my life. She has taught me so much about positive thinking, relaxation and finding that safe place in my life. It should come as no surprise that when I am looking for that safe place to go to, in my mind, I always chose the beach at Camp Ozanam. I spent 14 summers of my life there and shared my first passionate kiss with Jeannie on that hallowed ground.

As my relationship has continued with Betty over the years, it sometimes gets confusing. Is she my life coach or is she my friend? Which hat is she wearing? The answer is that she is a phenomenal human being whom I cherish and who will be part of my life forever. Thinking about her makes me smile and relaxes me instantly. I am a work in progress, but I am working. One of Betty's challenges to me was the need to keep a Gratitude Journal. We forever ask God for help, but do not take enough time to say "Thanks." Once again I am a work in progress. I go several days keeping the journal and then I get lazy. Life is all about choices. Make the time. In fact, when I complete this paragraph, I will make the time to write in the journal today – and Betty Leon will be at the top of the list today, followed by Jeannie, my kids, the other five "Rocks" in my life, and many of you! Betty has challenged me to follow the guiding principles of the Serenity Prayer: "God grant me the serenity to accept the things I cannot change, the courage to change the things I can and the wisdom to know the difference." Good guiding principles for all.

... *An Opportunity to Give Back*

In 2007, I continued to evaluate my life. Who am I? And where am I going? Those seem to be two questions that are fairly persistent. My family was growing – two kids were college grads. The business was not setting the world on fire, but was doing well enough. So I thought it over and decided it was time to give back to the community at large – time for volunteerism. The question was where. God sent the answer shortly thereafter. As I was reading The Branch from Our Lady of the Woods, there was an appeal from Oakwood-South Shore Hospital for help working in their Spiritual Support Department. As my mom was cared for at that very hospital and at the nursing home adjacent to that hospital, it seemed like the perfect way to give something back to the two places that took extraordinary care for my mom in her closing days. It seemed like a perfect fit. I went and "applied" for the job and was deputized. What an awesome ministry this is (it could be material for my 2nd book).

I typically visit between 25 and 30 patients each week. There are really two types of visits. The first type is that of a Eucharistic Minister. In that situation the main focus is to bring communion to the patient and their loved ones. Of course, many times more in-depth conversations follow. The part of the visit with their loved ones who are visiting is very important as they are often in as much need as the patient. Many times they are coming to grips with the reality that their loved one is preparing to enter into the next life, and I am proud to be able to walk that part of their journey with them. The second type of visit is referred to as a Day II visit. In this instance, I visit all rooms of people (no matter what their faith is) who are in the hospital for their second day. The purpose of that visit is to assess their needs for spiritual support. Many times those visits are short because there are no apparent needs. Other times the visits are lengthy, as years of concerns and questions are brought out. One thing is constant, God is always present. As I walk into each room I am meeting a stranger. I have no idea as to why they are in the hospital and what their spiritual needs may be. I pause briefly as I approach each room and I ask God to take over. He does! As I leave each room, I am sometimes amazed as to the nature of the conversation. I reflect and think, "I don't remember saying that", or "why did I say that?" The answer is simple – God put those words in my mouth. It is amazing what one can do when you turn it over to God. In many ways that is becoming more of a common theme in my life – quit fighting God for control and sit back and enjoy the ride. This is especially true of the recounting of my cancer ride to come.

Another benefit of this ministry is the relationship I have with all of the non-patients I come in contact with. The chaplains I have worked with, the other volunteers in the Spiritual Support Department, the doctors and nurses, the support staff (such as Housekeeping) are all a part of my day in the Hospital. My interaction with each of them also enriches my life. Truth be told, I get a lot more from my Hospital ministry than I put into it. It is the truth. I joined the staff to offer some help, but the patients and staff give me more than I give them. Thank you Lord for the gift of Hospital Ministry.

In June of 2008, we buried our friend and mentor from Burger King, Rod Jenison. Our restaurant was one of the restaurants Rod was assigned to watch over. He went on a phenomenal fishing trip with his sons. When he left he was not feeling well, but went anyway, as this was one of his life-long dreams. When Rod returned he was diagnosed with advanced pancreatic cancer and only lived a short time longer. We conversed several times on the phone, with me offering whatever encouragement I could. About a week before he died, I asked Rod: "Is there anything at all that I can do for you?" Without hesitating he said, "LOVE THE LORD!" Here the man was days away from his death and he is challenging **me** to Love the Lord. Those words will stay with me the rest of my life and I challenge all of you to follow those words as well.

... Ellen and Ryan Horner – November 19, 2010

Even as I type this I get a tad emotional. My daughter is married. When she was born all she did was cry. She was even christened, "The Soprano of Netherwood." At the age of five she got kicked out of pre-school. We knew we had our hands full. She was always in charge – she told Joey what to do (even though he was older) – hence she earned the nickname of "(Bossy) Boots." Her school years were actually pretty uneventful. Her favorite extracurricular activity was ballet. Even there she could be quite bossy as Miss Judy could testify. She was a great student and worked hard to accomplish any goal. The only goal she did not accomplish in High School was to go on "senior trip" because she had mean parents. Aunt Pat came to the rescue and bought Ellen a month in the tanning salon. Pat figured if Ellen couldn't go on "senior trip" she could at least look like it.

I can't comment much on her college years because she didn't live at home. Joe tried to celebrate her 21st birthday with her, but she was unavailable (the party started and ended early). It was a proud moment for her parents when she walked across the stage at Western. She got a teaching job at St. Stephen's in New Boston – and they are lucky to have "Boots" on their staff.

Ellen was always a social butterfly. But all of a sudden her life began to center around one man – Ryan Horner. The first two dates we were not allowed to meet Ryan, not sure why as I don't own a shot gun. Finally we beat Ellen to the doorbell for one date and met our future son-in-law. Their relationship has always been positive – they positively challenge each other's patience. In April of 2010, Ellen bought her house. From the time she announced she was house-hunting to the time of her purchase, less than a week had passed. It was her house. Not sure if that stimulated Ryan or not, but shortly thereafter we had "the talk." It was easy to give our consent. We did give Ryan one bit of advice, "sooner rather than later." Other than my own wedding and the birth of my three kids, Ellen and Ryan's wedding was the most joyous day of my life. We started out at 5:30 a.m. tailgating at the YMCA after Ellen's aerobics. And finished at 1:00a.m. at Malarkey's having an unnecessary "nightcap." I was denied permission to speak at the reception, but a bribe of the maître de gave me access to the microphone. I can remember how honored I was to *officially* welcome Ryan into the family. What the heck, he had been practically living with us for four years. I concluded my comments by asking everyone if they could "feel the love!" I could then and I can still feel it now.

My Children

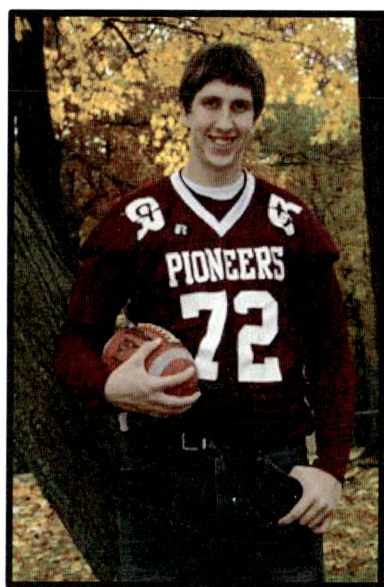

Matt's graduation picture

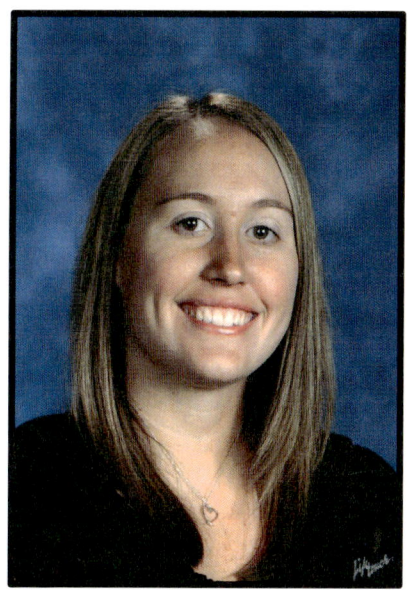

Ellen's school picture
2011

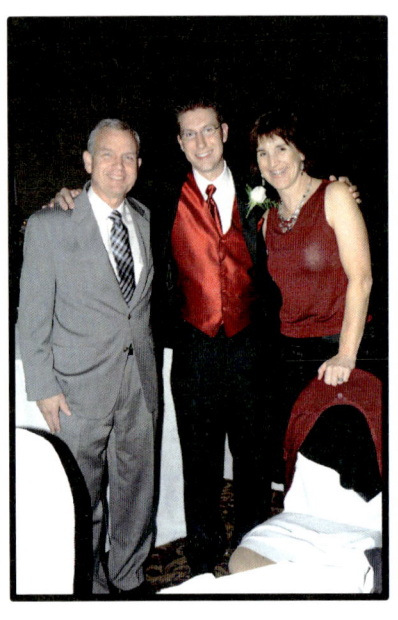

Joe with Godparents
Barb Koster and Kim Kiefer
November 19, 2010

Ellen and Ryan
November 19, 2010

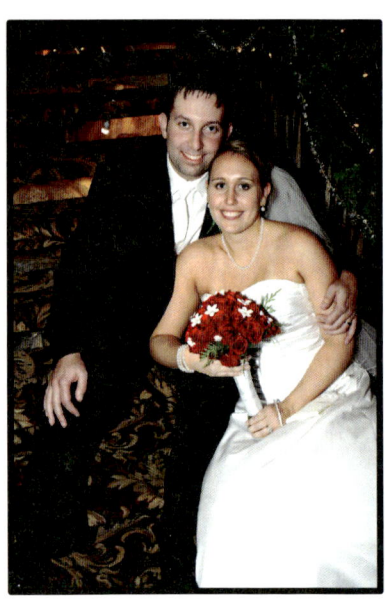

Chapter Two

2011
A Year to Remember

───────────────

... *New Year's Eve*

The older I get, the more sedentary I get. I can remember several New Year's Eve celebrations. Now I go to bed by 10:00 PM, and get awakened by one of the kids who want to greet the New Year. 2010 was not a bad year, but I always anticipate a better year to come. I gave up on the typical resolutions, but I do take some time to write down thoughts as to my expectations and prayers for the coming year. My dreams are actually not too complicated – protect my wife and kids is at the top of the list. Not too far behind is a prayer for the healing of the economy – for my business and for so many folks that are truly struggling. I am typing this in June 2011(?) and I still have those same dreams today.

Thursday, February 10th:

Joe's 29th birthday. I have decided to write about each birth family member as their special day crosses this time line. If there is ever anyone who has achieved the ability to always maintain a positive attitude it is Joe. I admire him for his ability to always be positive no matter what is happening in his life. Even as I type this I can hear his laugh and see his smile permanently affixed to his face. This year brought about more changes for Joe than most people see. He made the decision to end his engagement, he changed jobs, and he even had to move out of his apartment while waiting for the commissions from the new job to kick in. And all of this happened from half a country away in Las Vegas. He never called to complain. He just kept charging forward. A born salesman who is always positive. He is bound to succeed. I love you Joe!

... *Health Concerns*

Being a typical male, I do not place too great an emphasis on my health. Other than being overweight and a diabetic, I judge myself to be pretty healthy. 2011 brought some changes to that. I began to lose my appetite. Daily I would take some food to eat in the car on the way home. I began to be aware that most of the food that I was taking, I was throwing away – even a Whopper did not "hit the spot" anymore. But I thought it was a blessing because I was losing weight, an endless dream that I had for years. So there was no need to talk to anyone about this.

At the same time, fatigue was setting in. I began to challenge myself, wondering if this was what "old age" was feeling like. After all in October of 2011, I would be turning 60. I found an easy solution to curing the fatigue. Every day I would drive to work and go to the local "Park and Ride" and sleep however long I needed. People often complain that "nobody wants to get involved any more". I did not experience that. On at least three different occasions, some Good Samaritan pounded on my windows to make sure that I was OK. They saw me sleeping with the engine on. They wanted to make sure I was living. Yea, I was living; I was sleeping so that I could have some semblance of a distorted life. As far as the family was concerned, I was leaving for work at the same time every day. As far as the employees were concerned, I was just getting to work a little later. So there was no need to reveal my secret to anyone. I knew it would soon be over. At night I just went to bed earlier and so I successfully dealt with the fatigue. Pride can be a friend and an enemy–in this case it certainly was not my friend. By the end of January I was becoming concerned and had to share my secret with somebody. I had to swallow my pride (gulp!) and tell Jeannie what was going on.

Sunday, January 23:

I finally admitted to Jeannie that there was an apparent problem. The first thing in the morning the next day, I called and was seen by Dr. Nazareno. He was concerned about my symptoms and knew some tests had to be run ASAP. He arranged for me to go to the Southshore clinic and have blood work performed. This was not alarming at all because I go there once every quarter to have my diabetes monitored.

Wednesday, January 26:

I am still in a bit of denial and so this day Jeannie and I arranged to have a membership at Planet Fitness. Yes I was losing weight, so why not lose even more?

Thursday, January 27: Matt had a basketball game and Jeannie and I worked security. It is a good thing that GR kids and their fans are great, because we would not be a pair of guards anyone would want if there were any physical threat. I knew I was going for the blood work the next morning, which meant a night of fasting. I do not eat most nights, except when you know you have to fast and then I have a ravenous appetite.

Friday, January 28th:

The blood work was drawn without a hitch. I like to get there when the doors open at 7:00 AM. They took seven tubes of blood, three more than normal, but they were running some extra tests. Due to my lack of appetite, I was not famished as I usually am. I left Southshore by 7:15 to drive to the Park & Ride for my daily nap so I could be at work by 9:30. This was the new normal for me.

Monday, January 31st:

Time to take care of the mental and psychological part of my life. I arranged for a meeting with the afore-mentioned, Sr. Betty. I expressed my health concerns. She is always supportive and always challenging (some times more challenging than I would like her to be). She always ends our meetings with, "Love to Jeannie!" and off I went.

Thursday, February 3rd:

I am always practical and organized. I knew something was going on and so I wanted to have my life in order. That night we entertained our life insurance agent. I never told him my fears, but wanted to make sure that everything was well organized, and it was. He made some alternative suggestions about creative ways to pay the premiums. My mind was so preoccupied that I can admit I did not hear a word he said.

Sunday, February 6th:

A Super Bowl party at Ellen's. Once again I was so preoccupied that I cannot tell you who the opposing teams were, what Ellen served, who the other guests were (I do know that Brother Steve was there), etc. I know I was nervous about the test results and I was tired. We skipped the well-advertised half time show and I went home to bed.

Wednesday, February 9th:

I was spending too much time lying on the couch and was always cold so we had the living room measured for new windows, measured by yet another GR graduate.

Thursday, February 10th: Happy Birthday Joey – can my oldest son really be 29? Long-awaited appointment with Dr. Nazareno at 4:15 p.m. Of course, Jeannie went with me. Did she really think I would forget to tell her something? Dr. Nazareno glanced over the three pages of blood work. I am sure he studied them much more thoroughly prior to our arrival. I always look to the A1C number. It is a three month indicator of how well I am doing to control my diabetes. Lately my number had been slowly climbing, which is unacceptable. My one day fasting number was fine, so the day before I took the test I behaved, but the A1C number was not good. As the doc looked over my report, there were some numbers that were slightly elevated. Those numbers indicated that something was going on inside my body. That confirmed what we already knew. There was a reason for my fatigue and lack of appetite. Further testing was to be the next step. The good doctor arranged for me to have an ultrasound of the heart in his office the following Wednesday. He also gave me the phone number to a clinic to go for a CT scan of the abdomen. Dr. Nazareno is a much laid back gentleman. So the suggestion of neither of these tests alarmed me.

The clinic he referred me to is owned by yet another Gabriel Richard grad. It does amaze me how many places Gabriel Richard has infiltrated my life. I called the clinic and they had no openings until the following week. Then the scheduling clerk looked further and saw an opening for the very next day at 1:00 PM.

Friday, February 11th:

I arrived for the scheduled appointment and filled out the necessary paperwork. Filling out the same information for different doctors would become rather monotonous over the next few months. Now, I have mentioned that patience is not a recognizable trait in the Piotrowski family. I liked the 1:00 PM time frame because I figured I would be the first patient after lunch. Boy was I wrong. Even though Dr. Nazareno gave me no reason to worry – I did. How many times can you reread last October's People magazine? When I tired of reading I tried to nap, but was afraid to nap too soundly so as not to miss my turn. Lord knows I didn't want to stretch this visit out any longer. I kept smiling at the girl behind the desk, hoping that would help – it did not. Finally at 3:15 PM, I was called back. I was relieved. They put me on this table and began to take the CT scan, sliding me into this tunnel-like apparatus. I followed directions and was done in about 40 minutes. While I was getting dressed, the technician and the secretary worked on preparing a disk that would be given to me for future reference. This step figures later in the story. They presented me the disk and I was on my way to wait for the results and "enjoy" my weekend.

Saturday, February 12th:

I am the original worry wart, so what a better way to spend my weekend. What a waste of energy! But I am guilty as charged. TR has given me "worry beads" to help relieve the stress. The only thing the beads have accomplished is that I keep losing them, so I have to hunt them down, it keeps me occupied.

Sunday, February 13th:

A wonderful Sunday. The day began with our normal 8:00 AM Sunday liturgy at Our Lady of the Woods with Fr. Rick Macey. He truly is a wonderful pastor and has walked with me throughout this cancer journey. As is typical, we always go out as a family for breakfast after

Mass. It has been part of our family ritual. Another ritual/tradition that we have established is "Sunday supper." We gather together every Sunday for a family supper that usually includes Ellen and Ryan. It is a special meal. We gather in the dining room and use our "fine china." It seems that the only time that room and those dishes get used is on special events; only a few times each year. So we now make every Sunday special and it is the most enjoyable meal of the week.

Monday, February 14th:

Happy Valentine's Day, a day in which we celebrate love! I followed my normal routine. No breakfast. Left for work at 7:00 AM, drove to the Park & Ride for a nap, then on to Burger King for my work day, arriving at 9:30 AM. I never take the time to eat while I am at the restaurant. I left to go home around 1:30. I normally grab a sandwich for the ride home, but with no appetite there is no reason to eat; besides I am losing weight. On the way home my cell phone rings. A quick glance indicates that it is Dr. Nazareno. I thoroughly enjoy his presence. Before I answer, I know that it will be the doctor himself. He always handles these things himself, instead of passing it along to one of the ladies who work for him. In his typical "laid back" style, he informs me that he has the test results back from the CT scan and that he would like to see me as soon as possible. In that his tone of voice did not indicate any unusual problems, I pointed out to him that I was already scheduled to come into his clinic for an Ultrasound in two days on Wednesday, so why not wait. He said that would be fine. The Ultrasound was scheduled for 1:30 PM, so he agreed to see me to go over the test results at 1:00 PM. Because of some of the results from the blood work, I also had an appointment with my local "gastro" doctor the same day at 2:45 PM, so Wednesday would be a busy day.

Tuesday, February 15th:

I followed a regular work day; nothing out of the ordinary. When I got home from work, I had a discussion with Jeannie. She wanted to go with me for all of the appointments the following day. I told her that I was a "big boy" and didn't feel it was necessary for her to leave school early. Again Dr. Nazareno had not indicated anything out of the ordinary, I felt that I could handle whatever was ahead of me. Boy was I wrong! That evening we went to one of Matt's basketball games. It is so important to continue to support him and not let what was happening in my life take away from Matt and his aspirations. I went to bed and slept well uttering the Serenity Prayer as I often do when sleep is hard to come by: "God grant me the serenity to accept the things I cannot change, the courage to change the things I can, and the wisdom to know the difference." A true sign of things to come.

Chapter Three
An Alarming Discovery
Week One

Wednesday, February 16th, 5:30 AM:

Rise and shine. Watched Channel 7 Morning News. Is there ever any good news? Not normally. I began my normal work preparation.

7:00 AM:

Daily drive to Whitmore Lake.

7:50 AM:

Time for a break at the local Park & Ride; slept beautifully.

9:15 AM:

Arrived at work for a shortened day as I had to leave by noon to be at Dr. Nazareno's office on time. I am never late and proud of it. (Of course, now that I make that bold statement, I am sure my promptness will be suspect).

1:00 PM:

Arrived at Dr. Nazareno's office. One never has to wait at his office. His scheduling people never overbook and so you are always called back to the inner sanctum within minutes of arriving at his office. Dr. Nazareno always escorts you back himself. He sat on his little stool and I sat on the edge of the examining table, our normal positions. I started by expressing my concern about how long I had to wait for the CT scan, he listened attentively and agreed that the wait was excessive. Then he said he would like to go over the results. He literally read the report line by line. Being a professional hamburger maker, many of the words are not in my vocabulary, but the good doctor patiently explained everything to me. There were really three concerns indicated on the report:

#1. "Extensive diffuse fatty infiltration of the liver." In English that means that there is more fatty tissue on the liver than normal. Hmm. The doc explained that is really nothing to be concerned about. He said that with a change of my diet, eating less fatty foods and more foods with protein that problem can be easily corrected. I then talked to him about alcohol because I realized that alcohol gets processed by the liver. He said it would be a great idea not to consume any alcohol until this problem is resolved. He also asked what medication I took for the normal headaches. I told him that I am blessed in this area, but when I do take something I tend to take Ibuprofen. He strongly suggested that I stay away from this drug and he said to take Tylenol instead. No problem with that, other than I had just purchased a bottle of Ibuprofen and I can't stand to waste anything.

#2. "Projecting from the posterior aspect of the upper pole of the right kidney, there is a 2.7 x 2.5 x 3.3 cm enhancing mass identified. This is considered neoplasm until otherwise identified." Sounds like Greek to me. I asked the good doctor to explain. He said all indications are that renal cell carcinoma is present. Great! As stated earlier, I am a professional hamburger maker, so I now need an explanation of the explanation. Dr. Nazareno paused, looked me in the eye and said, "Chuck you have cancer." There was silence in the room. I digested his comment and did not know what to say. I looked at him and said, "Doc, did you just say I have cancer?" He confirmed my quick grasping of the obvious. I was speechless. I fought back the tears – I was going to be tough, but not really. I then asked, "How can they be so sure with just this test?" He responded that it is a strong indicator. There is nothing that it is 100% certain, but based on research and past studies, the test shows that I have cancer and he concurs with that analysis. Ouch! I then asked, "Is it treatable?" "Yes" was his quick reply. He went on to say that he personally, in his general practice, had not had an opportunity to deal with kidney cancer, but he would refer me to the best expert that he could find. He asked me if I knew of a doctor who had this specialty. I did not happen to have one in my address book. I then reminded him that I had been previously treated before at

U of M, where I had the Whipple surgery in 2004. I explained that I did not think the specialist who performed that surgery was an oncologist.

#3. Dr. Nazareno wanted to complete disbursing the information that he learned from the CT scan. He stated that, "In the superior left aspect of the L1 vertebral body there is a 2 cm sclerotic focus identified. Most commonly this would relate to a benign bone island." "There you go again, doc – give it to me in English." He rapidly stated that I had some kind of spot on my lower spine. He said that it was important to deal with the cancer right now and we would get to this spot later. It seems insignificant, but we sure would deal with it later, as you will see.

Dr. Nazareno left the room for an eternity – in reality was probably only about ten minutes. When he returned he handed me a one-page information sheet about Dr. Bruce Redman from U of M and told me to call him a.s.a.p.–a no-brainer for sure. In the ten minutes he was out of the room my mind went wild. I certainly could not pray that Serenity Prayer then, even though I should have. I realized that I could have had all of this information two days earlier had I chosen to come in when Dr. Nazareno suggested that he needed to see me as soon as possible. I got mad at myself and challenged myself why did I wait? The answer was simple. I wanted to economize on the time and, since I was already coming here for an ultrasound, what difference would waiting two days make? In the greater scheme of things, two days would mean nothing.

I want to digress here for a moment to tell you that one of the greatest lessons I have learned in this whole escapade is to react to any indication that something is out of the ordinary. I had been fatigued and did not have an appetite for a few months and I kept ignoring the symptoms. Duh – an illness is not going away just because you ignore it. **React as quickly as possible**. Doctors and modern medicine are really our lifelines. The true question is whether or not we choose to use them in a timely fashion. As I write this I have just gotten off the phone with Joe. Joe had just gotten off the phone with a friend of his whose father had just received the diagnosis that he too had kidney cancer. The problem with this gentleman is that he had some indications early on as well and he ignored those symptoms. He wrote it off to getting older and stress. His prognosis today was six months of life. My prayer for him is six months of peace. Six months to live life to the fullest. Six months not to beat himself up for not going to the doctor sooner. Six months to truly love his family and let them know. A few years ago we lost Rod Jenison to pancreatic cancer. From the time of his diagnosis until the time of his death he lived 27 days. He wasn't mad at God. And as you may recall, he was challenging me to "Love the Lord!" (AND ALL OF YOU), just three days before he died.

When Dr. Nazareno returned to the room and handed me Dr. Redman's information sheet, he inquired if there was anything I needed to know. I was still in shock and didn't know what to say. I asked about what courses of treatment were available. He repeated that kidney cancer was not his specialty. He was not aware as to whether or not radiation or chemotherapy would apply in this situation. He did make it clear that a person can live a full life with only one kidney, a fact that has been verified by countless people as they became aware of my condition. I was still numb, but knew there was nothing more that he could do. Besides I had two more appointments that afternoon. Life moves on. I did ask Dr. Nazareno, "How do I tell Jeannie?" He instantly volunteered that he would be happy to assume that responsibility. I told him that I didn't think it would be necessary. I told him I could handle it, but I told him to be ready for phone calls. Throughout my cancer journey I called Dr. Nazareno countless times for advice, information, support, and sometimes just to hear his reassuring voice. His support was invaluable.

1:30 PM:

Time goes on and I had an ultrasound scheduled in the room next door. I walked in and the cheery technician wanted to know how I was doing–under normal circumstances an obvious question. Today it was a tough one to answer. I had a huge lump in my throat. I calmly explained to her that I had just been diagnosed with kidney cancer and so it was not one of my better days. I went on to say that I was now extremely nervous about this test, worried (I told you I was a worry wart) about what other problems this test might uncover. She was very positive and upbeat. She told me that there is no necessary connection between kidney cancer and an ultrasound of the heart. The purpose of this test was merely to check on the condition of the heart. The test went off without a hitch. Of course, Mr. Impatient wanted to instantly know the results. The technician explained that she does not read the information. She would turn the results over to her superiors and somebody would be back with me in a few days. She sensed that I did not like her answer. Ding, ding ding! – right again. She repeated that legally she could not tell me anything. She then added that with all her experience she did not see anything abnormal with the analysis. Who needs a doctor when you have a supportive technician? Thank you, Ilana. I left that room knowing that I had no obvious heart problems. Dr. Nazareno did call a few days later to inform me that the ultrasound results were fine. I didn't bother to mention that I had been assured that a few minutes after the test.

2:00 PM:

I sat in the car for a few minutes, not sure what the next step was. I knew I had to make some quick decisions as to how to make the best use of these next few minutes because I had an appointment with my local "gastro" doctor. That appointment was set up before I was aware of the kidney cancer. It was set up as a possible source of information as to why I was fatigued and had no appetite. And, as I said earlier, I am never late. I knew I needed Jeannie with me. I called her and I told her that I was coming home to pick her up so that she could be with me at the next doctor's appointment. She laughed and mocked me. She reminded me that I told her I was a "big boy" and could go to the doctor appointments without her. She wanted to know why I had the sudden change of heart. I told her that I had time to kill so she might as well be with me. She said she would be waiting in the driveway.

2:10 PM:

Without realizing I was making a slight detour on my way home, the car drove itself to 2088 Tenth Street, the house in Wyandotte in which I grew up. I sat out front just for a moment and prayed. I had to get home and tell Jeannie the news that would change our lives. I began to organize my thoughts as to what I would say. I figured I needed some help. Sr. Betty Leon to the rescue. I called her and listened to her calming wisdom. To be honest, I cannot tell you what she said because I was so numb, but Sr. Betty is always calm and always wise.

2:25 PM:

There was Jeannie standing in front of the house with her customary cheery smile. I got out of the car and told her that I needed her to drive. She looked at me and said, "Chuck what is wrong?" *As I type this six months later, tears are forming in my eyes.* Despite what I had practiced on the way home, I looked at her and simply said, "I have kidney cancer." We wrapped our arms around each other and sobbed. I pulled away and told her we had to get a move on because I didn't want to be late for the next appointment.

3:15 p.m.

The doctor was late. Oh that is annoying. In this case it was fine because it gave Jeannie and me a chance to talk. Jeannie Byron Piotrowski is the most positive person on earth. From the moment she became aware of my cancer until her last breath on earth, Jeannie will not let adversity get her down. I gave her all of the details of what had happened earlier that afternoon. It did not and could not diminish her positive spirit. When we were finally seen by this doctor, he began to read my paper work. He started with the blood work. He began with a lecture about my elevated A1C count. I raised my hand and told him to stop and read on. When he got to the next page, he read of the kidney cancer diagnosis. He stopped instantly and said, "This is serious." Thank you Dr. Obvious. He said the rest of this visit would focus on treatment of kidney cancer – no more lectures about A1C. I explained to him that I would be obtaining the services of Dr. Redman. He felt it was obvious that I needed a little additional blood work, so he sent me to Wyandotte Hospital for those tests. Ten tubes of blood later, I was done.

4:15 p.m.:

Now how do I share this frightful information? I told Jeannie I would be strong and I would handle it. To start with I only needed to tell immediate family. I wanted to wait a few days for everyone else. Is this getting used to it?

4:30 PM:

We stopped at Ellen's house to tell her; phew! Nobody home. I am spared for now.

4:45 PM:

We arrived home and I could see Ellen was at our house. I would be able to tell Ellen and Matt at the same time. Of course, they had both been aware of my symptoms and were aware of the two doctors' appointments, so they were anticipating some new knowledge. I asked Ellen and Matt to sit on the couch. I figured I would tell them in the same order that Dr. Nazareno did. I started with the information about the liver. I told them that I had to eliminate fatty foods from the diet–lots of chicken and fish for the time being. I then added that I would not be drinking until this problem was resolved. Knowing what I was about to say, my eyes welled up *(they are doing that right now too)*. I looked at Jeannie and cried. I looked at the kids and said, "I don't know if I can do this!" Ellen, not knowing what I was about to say, rushed over and put her arms around me and said, "Of course you can do it." I gave her a puzzled look. She retorted that she knew I could eliminate booze and fatty food from my diet. I told her I knew I could accomplish that as well, but that there was more to come. She rejoined Matt and then I simply said, "I have kidney cancer!" Matt was the first one to burst into tears, joined quickly by the rest of us. We had a family group hug. Following the hug we had to clean up quite a pool of water. Jeannie took over and assured all of us that everything was going to be all right. As usual, she was so right. I was having a hard time believing it. I told the kids that, for now, I did not want to spread the news. Ellen wanted to call Ryan – her husband (still hard to believe that my baby girl is married). I told her that I would personally tell him. I felt that if people heard my voice they would know I was ok. I gave Ryan the prognosis and emphasized not to worry. The phone call with Ryan was hard, but it was getting easier each time I told the story. Completing the call with Ryan, I had to call my first-born son, Joe, in Las Vegas. In some ways doing this over the phone was easier because I didn't have to look at the person. In other ways it was harder because I could not reach out for a hug. Joe is a great hugger. He took the news in an upbeat way. Boy was the distance ever far that night. He wanted to know what he could do and I told him to pray.

The next person to tell was my mother-in-law, the original ultra-positive Jeanne Byron. She is one strong woman. I really hit the jackpot with Nonnie (her affectionate nickname). She assured me that I was fine and that God would be walking with me. Thank you Jesus! I then needed to call my mom's sister, Aunt May. She is a retired Sister of St. Joseph. I can still hear her saying, "Oh my lands" – an expression of amazement she often uses. Her spirituality is also quite deep. She assured me of her prayerful support and of the support of her entire community. Nothing like many nuns putting you on their prayer list. I am starting to lick this cancer thing already. One more phone call before the night moved on – Brother T. You already have heard how deep our brotherly relationship is. I knew I would struggle with this phone call. But it was easier than I thought. I had already explained my story a number of times so this was becoming a routine. TR said one thing, "I will be there for you." He always has and always will be.

7:00 PM:

Time to get on with living. Most people in the family were hungry. I was not. The consensus of the group was to go to Malarkey's; a fine Southgate establishment owned by yet another Gabriel Richard family. I know that the conversation was quiet and not sure if I even ate. I mostly just sat there and was getting used to the idea that I had cancer. In this infant stage of the disease it was still quite an obstacle. However, I would soon be able to say, "Surrounded by the Grace of God, WE Beat the Beast."

8:30 PM:

We got home and found Ryan sitting in the driveway. As he was supposed to be at work, this was a little disconcerting. Ryan explained that, after he talked with me, he could not concentrate at work. He explained the situation to his boss, and his boss gave him permission to join us. Only problem was that we were out pretending to eat. But Ryan obviously gets what family is all about. He was there to be together and help us, as family, to get through this obstacle. It was most appreciated.

10:00 PM:

It was time for the Fox 2 10 PM news – a nightly tradition, especially when my beloved Tigers are not playing, which is usually the case in February. Watching the news is never uplifting. To be honest, that night it was just some sound in the background. When the news was over we held onto each other so tightly. We had so many questions and no answers. Being in the early stages of cancer, I kept wondering "why me?" The answer is quite simple –"Because!" God does not have to explain anything to me. How many times in my life have I heard: "God doesn't give you anything you can't handle." In fact I am sure that I have used that line a few times myself. That night I was wondering the validity of that statement. Jeannie has always been most positive and was convinced from the first moment that we would get through it. At this point I was not so sure. I was the "doubting Thomas." We did not sleep too much that night. I went from the bed to the chair to the couch over and over again. How may infomercials can one watch in one night?

Thursday, February 17th:

Rise and Shine at 5:30 AM. Jeannie wanted to know if I wanted her to stay home with me. The answer was certainly yes, but I said no. I figured I had better learn how to lick this thing. Besides, I figured Jeannie would need to take some time off in the future–why use up those valuable sick days? I told Jeannie that there was no reason to keep this a secret so share away with the staff at school. She immediately went into Joe Whalen's office (the new principal) and gave him the news. He could not have been more supportive.

Thursday is my normal Hospital visitation day. I figured it was important to stick to the routine as much as possible. Sure would have been easier to feel sorry for myself and stay home, but what does that accomplish? We were slowly beginning to form a support group that is unbeatable. A support group that was surrounded by the grace of God and would give me all of the support that was needed. I decided that for today I would delay my trip to the hospital. I decided to start the day with Mass at Our Lady of the Woods. Our pastor is a pastor above all pastors, Fr. Rick Macey. He is the personification of compassion. To be honest, I do not remember what he preached about that day, but I know it was good. The importance of family is something I have heard Rick preach about any number of times (I think I was with Rick and his family on some of those trips to Buffalo) – a theme that is also important to me. After Mass, I asked Rick if I could talk to him. He changed out of his vestments and I met him in a darkened church. I could not hold back the tears as I gave him the prognosis. He so understood. He put his arms on my shoulders and broke into a wonderful spontaneous prayer. I took a deep breath and tried to relax. I felt better, but not cured. I went to the hospital and did my visits. I certainly had a different perspective about illness, as I was now one of them. I know I am a better member of the Spiritual Support team because of it.

I spent most of the rest of the day beginning to call my "family," my natural family and all of my extended family. Each call became easier to make and each call showed me just how powerful my family is. I was beginning to get off the "pity pot" and beginning to understand that it is possible to "beat the beast." I also sent a group email to my Sacred Heart Seminary family which I later copied to the rest of mankind. In my email to my classmates I stated: "We met because we all wanted to minister to others. We all realized the importance of prayer. Forty five years later we are all different (grown up?), but at our core there is still a relationship with God. I am asking that whatever form of prayer is prevalent in your life – USE IT NOW. Wednesday was my day to say 'life sucks' and I did. But the crying is over (mostly). It is time for me to realize that God is good and He has blessed me with a great life, an awesome wife, and three wonderful kids – and even a son-in-law that I really like. God will get us through this, but it doesn't hurt to pound the Heavens with our words." Boy, does the computer really accelerate communication. The computer is not the most personal, but it does get the word out in a hurry.

That evening I received an interesting phone call from Janie Gordon. Janie and I share one distinction; we are now cancer survivors. I met Janie in the early summer of 2009 on TR's pontoon boat, sharing a beverage, in the middle of Grandview Lake. (Isn't it amazing how often we gather together and share a meal or a beverage?) When I gather with TR and Janie and our families we always go to one of two favorite spots – TR's pontoon, which I just mentioned, or TR's Black Hole Tavern – the finest basement establishment at Grandview Lake. And the favored drink is Fireball, an exquisite cinnamon flavored whiskey -- yummy!) Janie is a bubbly person, filled with life. Her professional career is music and she always appears to have a song in her heart. Later that summer, we got the news that she had breast cancer. Our reaction was one of shock, just as the reaction of my family when learning of my kidney cancer. I can remember Jeannie and my praying for Janie on that same pontoon boat. She survived!! And now a little over a year later she called to offer her support. She said two things:

#1. "Have you gone online yet to get some information about kidney cancer?" I had to admit that just a few hours before I had actually done that. It was a frustrating experience, as the web site I initially found had so much medical jargon that I could not understand it. It was at that point I turned off the computer and decided I would only use the information from Dr. Nazareno and a team of specialists who would be mine. She then offered her advice; I needed to realize that this was MY cancer. There is no web site or book which will have the exact information for Chuck Piotrowski's cancer. "Own your kidney cancer!" I can still hear her making that exclamation. And that statement freed me up, I never returned to the internet.

#2. Janie shared with me an easy way to improve communication. There is a website called Caring Bridge (www.caringbridge.org) – as I write I will call this communication CB. The subtitle on the website states, "Connecting Family and Friends When Health Matters most." It sounds like a good place for me to end up. The purpose of this website is to be a journal. She explained that Jeannie and/or I could write a daily journal entry to keep concerned people informed. It was a ding…ding…ding moment. Already I have spent lots of hours on the phone and on the computer informing people of my dilemma. I realized that, as the process toward surgery continued, communication was vital. I also realized that there would be a time that I would not be available and all communication would become solely Jeannie's responsibility. This would provide all the "family" with up to the minute information.

The decision to use Caring Bridge was a real no-brainer. I knew it was another gift from God and I would work on setting this up throughout the weekend. Thank you Janie!

Who is God? An inspirational message I received taught me that our God empowers all without conditions of favoritism. Our God loves, forgives, and accepts us all eternally. Scholars and theologians could work to find flaws with this simple description. It is a description I lovingly accept. "Our God is an awesome God!" – Words to one of the many songs that I would repeatedly sing over the next several weeks.

February 18th:

The normal routine is followed. I went to the computer to check morning emails and spent much longer at the computer than I ever had. I could "feel the love!" My "family" was checking in for duty. The supportive emails were rolling in. Jeannie and I read them and cried tears of joy. Who had time to sit on that "pity pot?" We had work to do; we had to get on with living!!

I knew telling the Burger King part of the "family" would be difficult. I spend a considerable amount of time with them. I decided that I would opt to take the easy way out. I would write them a letter and post it on the bulletin board at Burger King. As I get older my handwriting is atrocious. Anytime I want my message read and understood, I have to type it. So I typed a note, put it in my brief case, and headed off to work. Due to the volume of emails and responses, I was quite a bit behind schedule–no time for the Park & Ride today.

I went to work and performed my morning routine and prepared the banking. I asked the restaurant manager, Eileen Contardi, to join me, something that I only do on rare occasions. Why should two of us go to the bank, when one can accomplish that chore? Eileen was antsy to know the results of the testing, as she had remembered that I had left early two days ago to get the results. Do you remember school days waiting to get the results of a test or a dreaded term paper? I sure do. As I described what I learned to Eileen, I followed the same format that Dr. Nazareno did. Start with the easy stuff. I can remember pulling into the bank parking lot and looking her in the eyes and saying, "I have kidney cancer." Her face registered complete shock and sadness.

She cried out, "Oh No." She put her head in her hands and sobbed uncontrollably. I told her that she had to see me as I told her so that she could see I was okay. In fact, she was the one crying, not me. By now I was used to the fact that these wayward cancer cells were growing in my body. She asked to stay in the car while I went in and made our daily deposit. I was not ready to share with the PNC family. One can only handle so much. On the way back to the restaurant, I told Eileen that I would be at Burger King as much as I was able to, but, for the next few months, my schedule would be dramatically different. She wanted to know how I would inform the rest of the staff. I told her it would be very emotional and I showed her the pre-typed memo. She agreed it was the best way to do it. My plan was to post the note and leave. I posted the note and stood back and watched one of my older and most loyal employees read the note. I could tell the exact moment that Chad learned of my fate. Is it ever awesome to have great employees? And I was leaving the restaurant in Eileen's capable hands. I had enough to worry about. Not worrying about Burger King with Eileen at the helm eased my pain.

On the way home I received a phone call from one of my lifelines, Rick Klapchar. Rick and I have been friends since 1965. We certainly have bonded in many areas of life, especially Camp Ozanam. We met at those precious 39 acres. His mom sent him to camp with a box of straws to use when drinking a pop. I mocked him and actually threw his straws all around the cabin we lived in. It's kind of embarrassing now when I realized how much Rick would walk with me during these next few weeks. Sorry Rick! Rick had read the email I sent out to all the classmates. Professionally, Rick is employed as a doctor at The Detroit Medical Center. He is the head of the Ears, Nose, and Throat department. But he knows a lot about everything. Of course, he was alarmed about kidney cancer. He was tremendously reassuring that it is beatable. He demanded that I carefully consider all options. He knew I was slated to go to the U of M and knew there were other options. He supported the option of cryosurgery. It was a term I had never heard of before, but one in which I would become quite familiar in the next week. I told him to send me an email explaining this procedure as I knew I would never remember all of the details. By the time I got home the email awaited. Cryotherapy "works well for tumors that arise on the outer part of the kidney and do not involve the urinary collection tubes." "Hooray!" I thought, this is me. Rick said this treatment is done as an out-patient procedure and done in the radiology department as opposed to the operating room. He has a personal friend who is an expert/pioneer in this field and he would be happy to set up a consultation. He ended his email with these comforting words, "Prayers and Blessings to you my good friend." Rick's wishes have been echoed by so many of you. I am in awe.

I did call U of M to set up my appointment with Dr. Redman. On their return call they explained to me that Dr. Redman had referred me to Dr. Hafez, whose specialty was kidney cancer. It was just a name to me at this point. It became a name that I will forever associate with the man who made me cancer-free. For this I will be eternally grateful. The appointment was set for Friday, March 4th, at 8:00 AM. Chronologically it was not that far away. Psychologically it seemed like a million years. I explained to the scheduling nurse that I was a tad anxious (REALLY) and that if there were any cancellations I could be there within thirty minutes. The nurse said that would be highly unlikely and that I should be happy to get in within two weeks. I was happy!

The emails and phenomenal support really started rolling in. It is overwhelming to feel that love. You always know that it is there, but when lots of folks take time to express it, words of appreciation cannot be found. This day I receive 35 personal emails – I normally don't get that many in a month. I need to make this apology right now I was thrilled to get every response that I received. I cannot possibly include them all. I have selected a few. I sincerely hope that if yours was not included that you are not offended. I just want to highlight a few:

From Elaine and Pete Simon (friends from St. Pius): Elaine wanted me to know that she prayed a rosary for me on the way to work. I was amazed that somebody took that much time to pray for me and I know that she has continued to pray that rosary daily.

From the Kulis (former neighbors), "all the good things you have done in your lifetime can now be counted on to get you through this."

From Tom Costello (cousin), "Good prayer, good care, and good attitude will get you through – I can't resist a triple play analogy.

From Greg Smykowski (friend), "YOU WILL NOT FACE THIS PROBLEM ALONE!"

From Greg Formella (classmate), "I anticipate a positive response."

From Andy Garlick (classmate), "I was devastated to learn of your medical challenge." *Andy sent several other messages, even one or two in Latin. Where is Fr. Walker when you need him?*

From Bill Bouie (friend), "Be strong my friend, you will beat this and we will laugh about this when we are watching the Tigers in the World Series this coming fall."

From Jim Stokes (friend), "I am sending positive energy. I have always carried you in my heart, now I will carry you in prayer too."

There are so many more, Yes, I can feel the love!!

February 19th and 20th:

My first weekend with cancer. I received lots of calls and emails and "well" wishes. I felt especially close to the Lord at Mass this morning. Prayer is good; therefore lots of prayer is even better. I have learned early in this process that it would be important to keep my mind active throughout this discerning process. One thing that I decided was very important was to set up the CB account that Janie Gordon suggested. For most people reading this story, it would be a minor challenge. For this computer-challenged Baby Boomer it became a weekend project. Once I began I was not about to let the computer win. Success finally came about 50 gray hairs later.

To begin CB you have to tell your story. I stated, "I received the word that I had kidney cancer on February 16, 2011. It was a total shock. Cancer is the scariest word in the English language. After about twelve hours of anxiety, I knew it was time to tap into the strength of my faith and my family and friends and conquer this beast!" Thus begins the legacy of CB. From this point on many of you will be helping to write this book as I plan to rely heavily on your words and Jeannie's and mine to tell this part of the story. One thing that I found interesting about my story above is that I unknowingly used the word "beast." It was the first of many times that I used this expressive terminology.

My brother TR and his wife Barb were in town for the weekend. We had a wonderful "Sunday supper" with them. It was a quieter setting. I can remember saying something silly to lighten the mood somewhat. I knew through this whole process, humor would play a tremendous part in reducing stress. Jeannie is a phenomenal cook and she gets better each year. But Sunday supper is also about the company present and the stories we share.

I received the first email of love from a niece or nephew. They are all grown up. It is incredible how many of them took the time to express their love and concern. I am so proud to call them family. Even as I write this I am smiling because they "get it" – they care and share. Today Katie Murphy emailed. She assured me that her whole family was on the prayer train. She included two Bible verses that have helped her in life. She was sure that they would fill me with the hope that only He can provide. They were:

Romans 15:13 "May the God of Hope fill you with all joy and peace as you trust in Him, so you may overflow with hope by the power of the Holy Spirit."

Phil 4:6-7 "Do not be anxious about anything, but in every situation, by prayer and petition, with thanksgiving, present your requests to God. And the peace of God, which transcends all understanding, will guard your hearts and your minds in Christ Jesus."

Monday, February 21st:

I received my first CB message; it was from my favorite daughter, Ellen. She states, "So glad I get to be the first to sign your guestbook… you know how competitive I am! While this may be an obstacle in your health, we know how strong you are and feel confident you will overcome it. God will answer our prayers!" *She is competitive for sure. One always prefers to have Ellen on their side.*

Tuesday, February 22nd:

I was very tired and so I decided not to go into work today. In the morning I emailed my buddy, Rick Klapchar. I told him that I had set up the appointment at the U of M. I further told him that I was very interested in also checking out this cryotherapy thing. The last statement I made to Rick was that I was somewhat anxious so I asked if he could expedite the process with getting an appointment at Karmanos. That email was at 6:15 AM and at 8:30 AM Rick was on the phone. He said he would do what he could to make an appointment. I told Rick I am available any time, get me in. It is amazing that in southeast Michigan we have two phenomenal options for treatment, U of M a leading research hospital and the Karmanos Cancer Institute; it is great to have choices.

At 11:00 AM, Rick called to say the specialist, Dr. Peter Littrup, could squeeze me in at 2:00 PM. Woohoo! It pays to know people in high places. I called Jeannie at Gabriel Richard (GR) and asked if she wanted to go with me. She immediately went to the principal and was given the afternoon off. That day we were having our computer worked on by a friend (Tim). He himself had kidney cancer over ten years ago. I explained to him the option of cryotherapy. He shook his head and said: "If it were me, I'd wanna get that sucker out." So now I had to start weighing my options and I hadn't even seen a doctor yet.

1:00 p.m.:

We arrived at Karmanos; what a huge complex. We began to fill out the first of a series of paperwork that it seemed like we did every time we went to a doctor. It is amazing how thorough they have to be, and most of it is to protect themselves from insurance companies. When we finished filling out the paper work in the admissions area, we were ushered to Dr. Littrup's office where we filled out the same paperwork, again. Then we were ushered into Dr. Littrup' inner sanctum and quizzed even further by Barb. She asked for the cd that the folks at the CT scan place had provided. She studied it for a few seconds and then informed me that the laboratory had sent the wrong cd. Not only did I have to wait forever, but then they sent the wrong cd. They have sent a cd of a chest x-ray that I had received ten months earlier. I was not a happy camper (LOL – the first time I attempted to type the word camper – I typed cancer' I guess my fingers type ca and they automatically finish cancer). Barb went on to say that Dr. Littrup would still meet with me, but would not be able to make a final decision as to whether or not I was a good candidate for this treatment until he saw the CT scan.

2:00 PM:

We began our meeting with Dr. Littrup. What an amazing gentleman. He spent more time with us than a doctor has ever spent with me in my life. He carefully explained his procedure and answered our many questions. Jeannie kept careful notes to which we would refer back. He explained that in cryotherapy he would take three long needles (the bigger the tumor, the more needles), penetrate the tumor and ablate it–freeze it to twenty degrees below zero. That would kill all of the cancer cells and it is less compromising of the kidney and its functions. The fact that I am also a diabetic always makes procedures a little more challenging. This doctor is a pioneer in this field and has done this procedure a couple of hundred times. It is done outpatient–in by 8 out by 3. I would have two or three days of discomfort, but then return to normal activity. There is not a 100% guarantee that the cancer will not return, but they would monitor me quarterly by performing a CT scan. Dr. Littrup urged me to keep the appointment at U of M; in fact, he used to work with the doctor at U of M.

Lots to think about, but being a wimp, I liked hearing things like outpatient treatment and two to three days of discomfort. I was convinced this was the way to go, but we have options. We did swing by Dr. Klapchar's office to thank him and he joined us for a Diet Coke in the lobby. Funny sidelight, with all of the scurrying around, I forgot to deposit the check to cover the payroll. So the payroll bounced, but the ladies at PNC who were members of my cancer support team, waived all fees. I did make a call to the place that performed the CT scan. They apologized and said they would provide additional CT scans as soon as their machine was repaired, which did happen three days later.

Chapter Four
The Band of Prayer Warriors Springs into Action
Week Two

February 23rd:

I posted an entry on CB that explained what I went through. Then I went to work. When I returned home I thought I would check to see if anyone signed my "guestbook" on CB. Up until this time the only entry was from competitive Ellen. I was amazed and overwhelmed to find 18 entries. I guess CB does work as a great communicating document.

J.R. wrote that he and Connie would be praying for me

Chuck and Jan challenged me to keep the faith.

T and Barb thanked me for having some encouraging words during Sunday supper that was "delish."

Even Jeannie wrote in the Guestbook and said, "I love you and know you will be healed. You are an awesome fella." *Thanks, Honey.*

Rita Costello was thankful that I would be going for a second opinion (guess I knew what she was thinking). She said, "Your faith and good attitude will take care of the cancer." Rita Costello was my mom. No, she is not writing me from the grave. Her sister is a member of the SSJ community of religious nuns. She is my Aunt May, yet most of the community knows her as Rita, because her professed name is Sr. Rita Agnes Costello–she shortens it to Rita Costello. So every time she sends me a CB message, it makes me smile as I know it is from Aunt May, but it makes me think of my mom.

My niece (Denise) wrote of her confidence that I would beat the beast. She said, "I love you tons." *What an awesome feeling.* She ended her message with "God Bless You."

Two of my sisters-in law (Cathy and Mary) wrote and used the exact same word, "encouraged." Their messages came 24 minutes apart.

Duke was a great friend throughout high school and college. He wrote, "while I don't possess the skill or power to lessen the uncertainty of the future, know that I stand with you, however dark the night or uncertain the path ahead."

I worked with Anne Michels in the mid 70's at Pat O'Grady's bar. She was forwarding my name to her church's prayer list (the more, the merrier). She thanked me for my "wonderful positive outlook" and challenged me to Stay Strong!

Joanne S. has two sons Jeannie taught at GR. She talked about how supportive Jeannie always was of her and now she is happy to return the favor.

Another sister-in-law (Pat) said: "It sounds like the good Lord is already at work for you. Praying for a positive outcome."

Frank & Kris assured me that I have an army of prayer warriors.

Donna Hughes told me to stay strong.

Tim Dombrowski is a priest friend. He gave me phenomenal encouragement: "You're in great hands with Dr. Littrup. He did his internship at St. Joseph Mercy Hospital, Ann Arbor, where I have worked since 1978. I had the privilege of reviewing some of his early research. He's a really nice guy!" *Now there are two good friends singing Dr. Littrup's praises.*

Peggy (sister-in-law) is continuing to pray. I have a total of eight sisters-in-law; glad they are all on my side.

Andy continues to support me.

Theresa Howard said that she would "Journey with you in prayer." *It truly is a journey with an unknown itinerary.*

Thursday, February 24th: My entry for the day centered on my concern that I had a lack of energy. The cancer was zapping me daily. I napped an awful lot. I was looking forward to the U of M appointment so that I could weigh both options and decided which path to follow. "I had thought about Easter vacation or summer vacation for the surgery, but that would not work. The waiting would drive all of us nuts. I did want to make it clear that I was 100% pain free, which was awesome. Keep praying and believing."

Joe Whalen (GR principal and friend) "Fight the good fight, Brotha. We need you in the stands cheering on those Pioneers! We're behind you and your family, just like you are always there for us."

Anne and Paul write: "We like the Karmanos option. It's very good to get that second opinion also, especially from U of M doctors. We look forward to a long wonderful relationship with both of you."

Pete and Elaine: "This burden shared by the ones who love you is just a fraction of a burden... the joy shared when you win will be a tsunami of joy. Keep laughing. You are always in our prayers."

Joan Walsh (a great friend who has had many cancer struggles of her own): "So glad you went to Karmanos – that's where all my angels are and where I had my treatments! U of M is where I had my surgeries – you'll be in excellent hands wherever you end up. You are in our prayers and through our prayer chains all over. Wishing you peace, now that you are moving forward with consults and plans – I know the "unknown" and the "waiting" is the worst".

Jeannette Frasson (another great friend who has beaten cancer six times to date): "Chuck, the big C can be beat and/or put on the back burner for a long, long time, I'm proof of that. And I'm confident that you'll be beating it too! Keep that positive attitude; it does make all the difference. God Bless you!"

My cousins Mickey and Chris commented on the greatness of modern medicine and are praying for me.

It is humbling to know how many people are praying for me and including me in various prayer chains – little ole me. In addition to the prayer, positive attitude and laughter seem to be common denominators.

Barb Koster said, "You ARE going to beat the beast. You have such a positive attitude and outlook. Much love and many prayers."

Isn't love grand? I feel so many people wrapping their arms around me and giving me a great big squish. I know I will always challenge myself to express that love that I feel. Hugging is great. Saying I love you is even greater. And today is Ron Victor's birthday.

February 25th:

My journal entry: "Good morning and congratulations to all of you school employees who have managed to gather up yet another snow day! The doctor's report was very encouraging. On the day I was first diagnosed with cancer, they took 10 tubes of blood for additional testing. They tested for every kind of cancer imaginable. Every one of these tests came back NEGATIVE. So the only cancer is that silly three centimeter tumor on the right kidney. The doctor also was thrilled that the ultrasound of the heart came out victorious–even though some of you have accused me of being heartless! Dr. Nazareno explained that he does not have knowledge about the cryotherapy option, but he would get more information. He did offer his concern about my body if surgery was performed and the kidney removed. Yes, one can live with one kidney and do it very well. In my case, however, being a diabetic and having high blood pressure would require a stricter routine to make sure the remaining kidney would not be compromised, but still very DOABLE. To be honest, the prior day was a tough one and I was not sure why. I allowed the "stinkin thinkin to enter my feeble brain and so I was stressed all day. Lots of pain in the upper back, at times unbearable. But I had a nice hot heating pad and some ibuprofen and I woke up the next morning pain free and ready to take on the day."

Barb Koster was glad to hear I was pain free, but concerned that I not shovel the snow that caused the snow day. She laughed about Ellen getting a snow day because the day before Ellen stressed about whether or not she would get a snow day. Ellen was not sure if anyone knew the proper call-in code. (I think Ellen called it in herself.) Barb closed with "stay warm." *I am so warm and fuzzy because of my wonderful support system.*

Mary Kuli wrote: "God Bless you, Jeannie, and the kids thru this trying time. Thank Our Dear Lord for our Faith! Hang in there and let's all keep praying!"

I have often wondered throughout this time what do people do who do not have faith?! Where do they draw their inner strength from?

The Chircos (St. Pius friends) said that I have a heart of gold, no matter what anyone says. "Please continue to keep the faith as we know that you and the Good Lord will always prevail."

Aunt May: "So many decisions for you to make. I am sure the Dear Lord will guide you when you have all the facts to evaluate. I know for one I have placed both of you in the hands of the dear Lord that I know you can't go wrong with your decision."

Saturday, February 26th: I wrote about events from the previous day. I had mailed the correct disk to Karmanos to review my CT scan. I wanted to make sure they received the disk and wondered if they had a chance to read it. Barb answered the phone on the first ring. "I identified myself and she instantly said, "Hi Chuck, I was just looking at your disc that came in the mail today." I never expected to get a live person, have her know who I was, and know what I was calling about. They really seem to care about the individual. Caring about the individual is what life is all about, whether it is one of our kids, a coworker, or a complete stranger that we might be able to help. I love the action described as "a random act of kindness," unfortunately, I do not do it often enough. Thanks to all of you for all of your random acts of kindnesses directed to me. We are all in this together."

Patsy (my favorite sister): "Sending love and beautiful morning Light from Vermont to you, Chuck and Jeannie. We will use this link as a way to stay in touch as you take the next steps in this process. All our love."

Rita Costello (*I do enjoy typing that name – Hi Mom!*): "The sisters look forward to your updates since I post them on our Bulletin Board. This really keeps them informed plus the prayers going your way. Be good to yourself and take the rest. They say rest is the best medicine." *What a great feeling to know that I have all of those sisters praying for me. They are professional pray-ers; and after all those years of praying, I know that God hears them loud and clear.*

Gwen (my niece-in-law's mom), *the family keeps growing – the more the merrier*: "With the strength of your family and friends you will make it through, we are all here for you and pulling for you.

Barb Koster: "Take it easy! If your body says "REST" then rest and don't worry about it!! And WE will all keep praying.

Theresa (another SSJ) is still praying and reading the updates.

TR *(you already know what a special brother he is)*: "God gives us challenges to make us stronger. You will beat this cancer. You are my HERO!!! Get well – we are going to Vegas!" *This is one of the more humbling statements. I do not think I can be a Hero. Yet TR has designated* me that and continues to use that term. I am not worthy, but hope to be able to live up to that. It's especially moving that he commented because he is not really into the computer, so I am honored that he, too, as so many others, was following along.

Sunday, February 27:

In my Journal I wrote: If Patience is a virtue; Jeannie and I are virtue less. This waiting is numbing, but we know there is nothing one can do about it. How many times have I said, "Why me?", since the <u>C</u> word crept (or slammed into our lives). Mornings are the time with the most energy – hence the earliness of these postings (4:15 AM) There are three church songs that I sing or hum several times each day: "Be with me Lord when I am in trouble!," "Our God is an Awesome God!," and my favorite, "God Has done Great Things for us, filled us with laughter and music!" The first one is to ask God for His help and guidance and the other two are to always praise God because He is awesome and He blesses us with all things that are good! The last verse I also used six years ago as my mom was dying and we sang it at her memorial service.

Hope you all have a wonderful Sunday and an even better "Sunday supper" – a Piotrowski tradition."

Today I received a phone call from Jay Yule, a lifelong friend. He and I attended High School together. In our first year of college, we shared a room together with Andy Garlick and Bill Koviak. I think we drove the latter two nuts as they moved out before the end of the year. We ended up working together at Camp Ozanam, and we ended up working together at Pat O'Grady's Bar (…I will leave up to your imagination as to which of us actually danced on the bar to <u>You Make Me Feel Like Dancing</u>). Jay was one of the earliest walkers in this cancer journey. And when you walk with Jay, Mary and the kids (Sarah, Tim, and Dave) are right there with you. I am not the greatest texter, but throughout my cancer journey, Jay and I often sent a quick text during the day. Jay's positive outlook and sense of humor helped pull me through a number of times.

Speaking of phone calls, I also heard from my son, Joe, today. Several months ago Joe decided to follow his dream and move to Las Vegas for the next stop on his life tour. There sure have been some challenges for him, but through it all Joe has maintained a positive outlook. I have never heard him negative or ready to throw in the towel. Joe truly believes in living for the moment. I admire his positive attitude so much. And it is this positive attitude that Joe has used daily in his phone calls to support Jeannie and me. The physical distance is a real challenge. I know he will not be physically with us as I undergo surgery, but his heart will be right there and I know he will be one of the last people I call before surgery. Joe's daily calls are always uplifting and today's was no exception.

There were two entries on CB today. Both my aunt (Rita Costello) and my sister-in-law (Pat Gonyea) expressed similar sentiments. They talked about five more days of waiting before the appointment in Ann Arbor. Pat commented that I inspired her. Every time one of my "walkers" tells me that, I am humbled. I never set out to do any inspiring. I started this CB as a way of journaling what was going on in my life and in my mind. I always honestly express what is on my mind; some days you get grumbling, but most days you get a positive outlook which is fortified by the knowledge that God is with me. And, as I have written earlier, one of the ways I reinforce God's presence is to sing different church songs that convey some powerful sentiments. It is no wonder that Pat ended her entry by saying, "keep singing." And my dear aunt wrote about the need for patience: "The waiting game is always the hardest. If I know what I am handling, I react much better. To wonder what the second choice might be requires patience."

Monday, February 28th:

In my journal today I wrote that we are in a holding pattern until U of M on Friday. Rick Klapchar came through again. A personal friend of his actually had the cryotherapy treatment a year ago. Rick will put me in touch with the gentleman. I will learn what he went through then, and how it has changed his life.

I continued, "Thanks to all of you for your thoughts and prayers. When I went to the bank today, the manager gave me a refrigerator magnet. It had a quote from Winston Churchill: "Never, Never, Never Give Up!" And we won't until the beast is gone and forgotten."

Gary Zilli (classmate) *as I typed classmate after Gary's name and several others it occurs to me that it comes across as somewhat impersonal. Class mate is how we met, but lifelong friendships are present in many of these relationships* wrote: "One thing that came about strong in your message about your health is your faith, hope, and love in God. As His disciples, we know that He is with us, and in us, always. His love and mercy for us is beyond description. Like you said, He is an Awesome God." *Gary went on to offer his help to do any running around that anyone in my family needed. It is an offer that so many people have made – an offer that we do appreciate. Gary is a retired parole officer and now spends a lot of his time volunteering at St. Sylvester's in Warren, pastored by (you guessed it) another former counselor from Camp Ozanam, Gary Schulte.*

Anne Michels says, "So very true, NEVER GIVE UP!!!!!" You and yours continue to be in my prayers. Friday will be extra, extra prayers… Continue to stay positive." *Anne ends this entry as so many of you often do with xxoo – I have never been hugged and kissed so much in my life – keep 'em coming.*

Aunt May reminded me that the love of family will pull me through the four days before the conference at U of M. She has spoken to my cousin Lynn MARIE and I have the support of that branch of the family. *What is family? In the biblical sense we are all brothers and sisters. And through my cancer journey I have lost count of how many brothers and sisters I have. Praise God for presenting me with such a large family!! Lynn's dad had a closed head injury a few summers ago. George was my godfather and a special man. His life philosophy was that if you weren't having fun, what was the use of doing it?! What a way to live life. It was my privilege to walk with George that last summer of his life. I especially enjoyed the times I was in his room all alone while his kids went for something to eat. I could tell him how much I loved him; even though I was not sure he could hear or understand me. I wish I could be half the man he was. His funeral was on October 25th, my birthday – how appropriate. God Bless George, Lorraine, Lynn MARIE, Mary Jo, Tom, and all of their families.*

The last CB entry for today was from a complete stranger, Camille Demario. She is a former SSJ and a great friend of my aunt's. My aunt told Camille of my plight and she decided to walk with a complete stranger out of respect for my aunt. She has kept us in prayer. I am in awe. *Out of complete coincidence I had the pleasure of meeting Camille later in the year on June 22nd. As I hugged her it was as if I was hugging a life-long friend. Thanks for walking with us, Camille.*

March 1st:

I wrote, "Where did February go? Good riddance I say. I did have quite a phone conversation with Jim yesterday. Jim is a **kidney cancer survivor.** He is an ENT doc at DMC. He had cryotherapy a little over a year ago. He called his decision to undergo this path of treatment a "no brainer." He is a tremendously upbeat person who certainly understands the challenges of cancer. Before making his decision he did a lot of research on both the treatment and the doctor performing the surgery, and you can bet his research was a lot more thorough than mine. He is convinced that Dr. Littrup is the leading doctor in the US, if not the world, to treat cancer this way. All good news to me. Jim had the treatment on Thursday and was back to work full-time on Monday morning. Jim could not rave enough about how simple the treatment was as opposed to the major surgery of removing the kidney. Jim was also concerned that, being a diabetic, my organs already do extra work before eliminating the kidney. If you have to get cancer good to do it in southeast Michigan with Karmanos and U of M in our backyard – and with the leading cryotherapist in the US at Karmanos. Our appointment is Friday at U of M. Will be great to get that "second opinion" and then be able to make a well-informed decision. Thanks for your love and support." *To be honest, I have not verbalized this to Jeannie, but I am convinced that this is the way to go. Jeannie, on the other hand, favors the U of M option, even though it has not been formally presented. One thing we have in common is that it is* securely in the Lord's capable hands – He will guide our decision.

Aunt May wrote, "Jim's input sounded great, very encouraging. I am still happy you are waiting for a second opinion. The second option came into our lives for some strange reason. With the help of the dear Lord, you will make the right decision. I'm also asking your dear mom (the real Rita Costello) to intercede on your behalf."

Barb Koster says, "Wow!! What an encouraging story! Back to work in three days. I know you'll be glad when Friday comes – at least now the appointment is this month!"

Peggy (Jeannie's sister and my friend) told me all of the words in today's posting are encouraging. *Encouraging seems to be the word of the day – a pretty good word to have.*

Frank and Kris (good friends from St. Cyps): "You continue to be in our prayers, but every post you make sounds more and more upbeat and confident. We're hoping your visit to U of M makes your final decision an easy one ... one you will believe in your heart of hearts and then on to the next step…winning this life interruption."

My "Rocks"

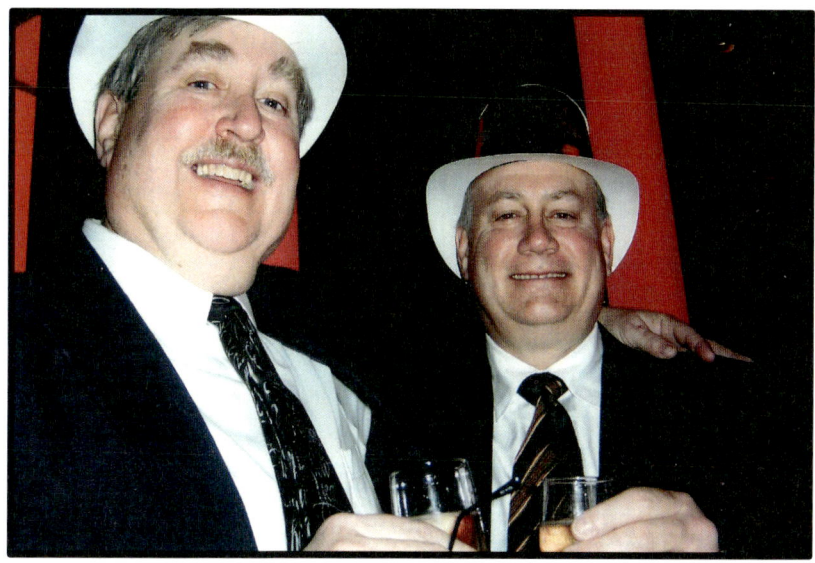

Chuck and TR

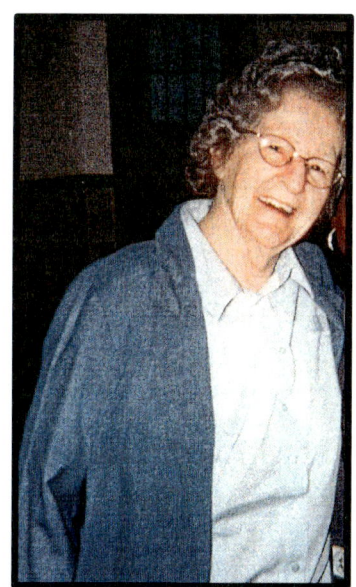

Sr. Mary Finn, former professor

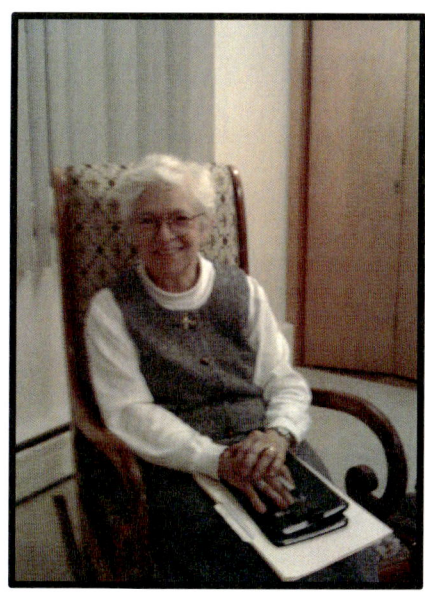

Sr. Betty Leon

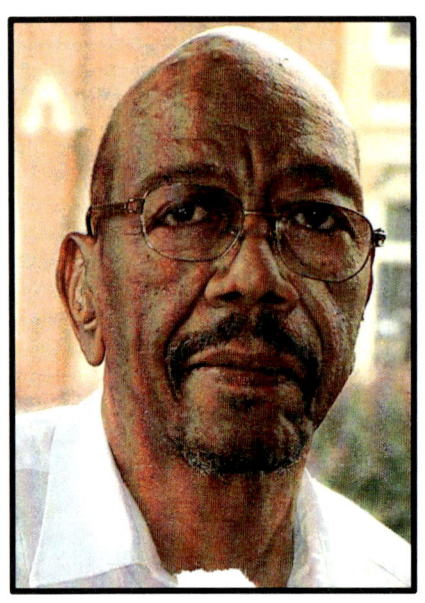
Mr. Jerry Brown

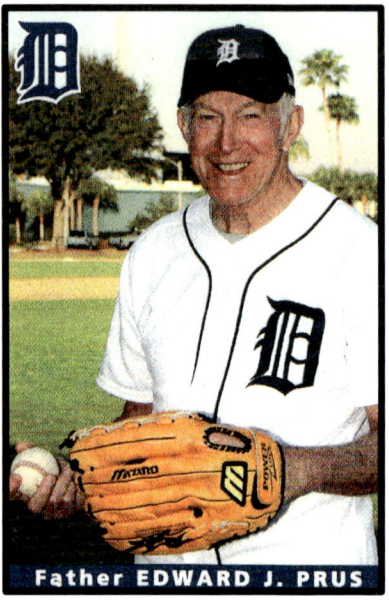
Fr. Ed Prus, former professor

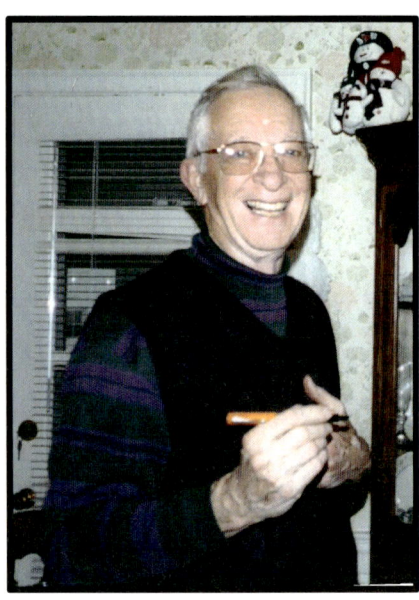
Uncle Earl Loeffler

Chapter Five

Decision Making
Week Three

March 2nd:

Hard to believe that I posted nothing for this day. But looking back, with the appointment at U of M just two days away I was preoccupied and probably decided not to share my anxiety with anyone today.

My aunt (my personal prayer warrior) wrote that she was impressed with what is taking place to help me come to a right decision. She reminded me that God is with me and pronounced blessings on me and my day.

My niece Jane Maxwell with her husband and two (soon to be three) sons have been walking with me throughout. Today she wrote three words, "We Love You!!" *I cried then and I cry now.*

Joan Walsh (fellow cancer survivor) sent lots of love and prayers. She said "only one more day of waiting. Glad you will be able to make a decision as to medical facility and be able to be ready to attack that tumor."

Theresa Howard commented that her sister currently goes to Karmanos for treatment. Theresa goes with her for treatment and likes the atmosphere. "Praying all will fall into place."

Gwen D. continues to walk with me. She is amazed by my strength and courage. She says I am an inspiration to the folks reading CB! *I don't deserve the credit people give me for being positive and having courage. I thank everyone for those comments. I just choose to focus on more positive things; and when I have a bad day, I omit the comments or sugar-coat them. When I was in college, Ron Victor and I went to Hazel Park race track more than we should have. When we won, we couldn't get back to the seminary fast enough to brag to our buddies. In fact we missed one Easter Vigil due to the alluring ponies. We snuck in the back door and didn't even admit to going, but Sr. Mary Finn looked at me and smiled (she knew). Hence it is easy to write about positive days and sweep the other ones under the carpet.* Gwen concludes today by promising to send positive energy every day.

I guess this is a great time to talk about Ron Victor. He is another seminary friend for life. We also met in 1965. Together we have shared so very much. He was much brighter than me so his help came in handy more than once. We actually took a class together, in which we were the only two students, Historiography which met at 7:00 AM. The prof lectured from notecards which were written in German, but he spoke in English.

Gambling is a common pleasure. In addition to the race tracks, Ron and I have been to Vegas together and, not too long ago, Jeannie and I were at MGM casino and looked up and there was Ron playing video poker. I was thrilled to have been asked by Ron to speak at his ordination celebration. Then I realized I had to actually say something. I was inspired to talk about Ron Victor as a man with extreme faith and he still is!

Thursday, March 3rd:

"Today the phrase, "the triumph of the spirit" is dominating my thinking. Is it really as simple as that? Of course, we humans always complicate things. Since my diagnosis, last night was the first time I have slept through the entire night. WOOHOO! And I certainly am not getting used to cancer; it is "the triumph of the spirit." The C word is scary, but not the end of the world for all of us. My buddy, John, has had cancer for several months – his treatment plan is in place, but he cannot go for surgery until April 17th and the passing of the tax deadline. Then there is the story of Kyle, a 20 year old GR grad. He is dealing with Hodgkin's lymphoma. Pray for both of them – it is not fair for anyone, especially a 20 year old. And each of you could add ten names of your own to this list. The triumph of the spirit also comes into play. Since I believe in endings, I know that **there are only happy endings.** The other day at a Burger King meeting somebody wanted to know what kind of diet I was on. I looked at him and said, "Cancer" – and I could actually chuckle. No, I am not getting used to it. We went to a GR basketball game last night and one of my buddies was surprised to see me there. Did he think I belonged home in bed? I have to get out and get support from all of you, support whether or not the people I am with even know I have cancer. As humans we are not separate individuals, we are all connected–thank God! Thank God again for all of you and your support.

Aunt May wrote: "One more dark day and you will know the second half of the evaluation which will be most helpful for you to make a decision. I am proud of you for dealing with this cancer. *(Did I have a choice)?* You and Jeannie have great faith for God but also for each other. May the dear Lord continue to bless you and guide you through your final decision."

Bonnie DeMeyere is one of those life-long friends. We worked together at Camp in the 70's. We go several years without talking, but then pick up right where we left off. She learned of the cancer and contributes to CB. "I was encouraged by your visit and procedure from Dr. Littrup. And then further backing from Dr. Jim who is a success from it! Any time you can keep your organs, prevent major surgery, and still have a successful outcome, that's a plus." At the conclusion of this entry she was leaving on a ski vacation. *Can broken bones and cold weather be a vacation?* She assured me of long distance prayers and thoughts throughout her vacation.

Tonight I received an awesome phone call from my friend Cliff Moening. Cliff and his wife, Ruth, are faith-filled dynamic friends from St. Cyprian's. We have been to several parties at their home and are pleased to share a joyful life with them. Cliff was made aware of my kidney cancer diagnosis. Cliff himself had kidney cancer in January. He wanted to call and share with me what his course of treatment was. Cliff was treated at the main Henry Ford Hospital. The course of treatment he received was to have the kidney removed robotically. Cliff could not emphasize enough what a painless and efficient procedure it was. Cliff had the tumor removed on Thursday and was home and comfortable, following a normal routine on Monday. He just wanted to share his optimistic path of treatment. Of course, Cliff is always optimistic, one of the most optimistic people I know. I appreciated him presenting yet another option to me. What to do? Cryotherapy? Robotic therapy? Removal of the kidney? All good options – I will continue to collect information and make a wise choice that works best for me. *On a sad note: Cliff recovered fine from kidney cancer, but a few months later, he encountered a brain tumor- which claimed his life on August 17th, 2011. I am a lucky man to have had the privilege of knowing Cliff and the honor to call him my friend. Rest in Peace, Cliff!*

Friday, March 4th:

"We're off to see the Wizard…" "Other related thoughts to that movie: 'There's no place like home;' from another song whose name I don't remember, "Oz didn't give nothing to the Tin Man that he didn't already have!" – a big heart!! My favorite tie I own was given to me 30 years ago by my godson (Tim Yule)–Mary probably bought it and never took the credit. Anyhow it is a tie with pictures of the Cowardly Lion throughout the tie–the King of the Kingdom. I still wear that tie and absolutely love it.

This is the day we have been waiting for and it's a typical March Michigan winter day. Coming from the east, the drive was not bad. We got to the hospital at 7:15 for an 8:00 AM appointment; I hate to be late. We got the very first parking spot in the garage, unusual. Walked into the hospital and wondered if we were in the right place, it was empty. Got on the right floor and many of the reception areas still had the partition screens down. Something was not right. This better not be a bad early April Fool's joke. As it turned out, people who were coming in from the North were stymied by some of the worst icy roads. Being a Friday, many folks had already called off. The lady we talked to said it took her three times as long to get in. Once again I was given the ever-familiar clip board so that I could record all my medical information for the new doctor. I should have just run off copies. Upon completion, the nurse weighed me and took all kinds of other information. I was then ushered into the examining room. The nurse who ushered us in said that she knew the nurse who normally took the next step was not coming in. In fact, due to the treacherous weather, the nurse wasn't even sure if Dr. Hafez would be in. Ouch!

She called around and, sure enough, Dr. Hafez was in the house and would be with us shortly. A short time later he appeared and the next chapter began.

Dr. Hafez began by giving us a brief history of U of M's involvement with cancer. The wing that we were in is seven stories high. The first two are reserved for testing and patient visits. The top five floors are totally dedicated to research. Over two-thirds of this massive structure is for learning purposes, which is amazing. In fact, Dr. Hafez's business card lists him as a Professor. We had to inquire to make sure that he was actually a doctor, for peace of mind. We had earlier done research on the good man on the Internet so we knew he was a certified doctor, originally from Egypt.

On CB I wrote, "Well there was a stop light half way through the yellow brick road; a very long day and more questions than answers. I was very impressed with the U of M doctor. He spent a good hour with us. Unfortunately he is at the other end of the spectrum from the Karmanos doc. Karmanos says do not consider surgery, do cryotherapy. U of M says do not consider cryotherapy, you have to do surgery. What to do? There are three options for the surgery. In all three cases they feel they would only have to remove 25% to 33 % of the kidney along with the tumor. They would prefer to do open surgery in which they would go through the back which would not disturb the chest cavity which had already seen the Whipple surgery six years ago.

Dr. Hafez looked at the old CT scan from six years ago and the tumor was already there. It was only a centimeter and was easily overlooked, but now Dr. Hafez knew where to look. He figured it had been growing for ten years. That being said, the doc is also very encouraged by robotic surgery and its success. With robotics, they would go through the chest cavity, but would only need six small pinholes, no cutting (which is an obvious advantage). The doc said he would like his team to review my situation and come to a consensus (are they voting on my guts?) as to which treatment plan would work the best. Complete recovery would be up to six weeks. *Huh, as I type this we are at three months and we are not close to complete recovery – I guess they count different or give you the best case scenario while you are pondering a decision.* I could drive as soon as I would be off all pain medication. Hospitalization would be three to five days. The doc did caution us that if the kidney has excessive bleeding during the surgery, there would be a chance they would have to remove the whole kidney.

I talked to the doc about the problem I was having with fatigue, weight loss (25 pounds in six weeks), and a CEA number (not sure what it is) being elevated. I told him the other docs all agree that those factors have nothing to do with the cancer. This doc agreed. In fact he was downright concerned and annoyed with my local gastro doc. He said there is no way he would even consider surgery until he knew what was causing those other problems. He recommended a U of M doc, Dr. Thomas Wang, to run additional tests to discover what was causing those problems. He also strongly recommended that I not go back to Karmanos until we had the results of Dr. Wang's tests. So we made an appointment with Dr. Wang. The earliest we can get in is March 25th, three weeks from today. We asked Dr. Hafez to put pressure on Dr. Wang to move up that date. The best they could do was to put us on a cancellation list. We told them we could be there within an hour any day of the week--very disappointed and frustrated. Thought we would have a more defined game plan to deal with the cancer. But the route we are going does make sense and I am OK with that. Thanks for walking with me.

Bill Brazier wanted to sing a Camp Ozanam song. As you know, I spent 14 summers at Ozanam and worked a total of 30 years for St. Vincent de Paul Society. The song lyric that came to mind is, "It's a name that a shame never has been connected with." Wouldn't that be a nice thing for any of us to lay claim to for ourselves? Guess I have some work to do.

There were eight responses today on CB, including Bill Brazier's (executive director at St. Vincent's).

Aunt May wished me well and commented: "You are at U of M waiting your turn. I'm on the way to chapel for your intention. The yellow brick road is now coming to an end in one way."

Camille wrote, "May your yellow brick road bring you

enlightenment and peace of heart, as you embrace your road of decision. My prayers for you and your family." *It is important to remember that the ultimate decision may be mine, but it is paramount that I consider the feelings of Jeannie and the kids.*

Niece Denise wished me luck and is praying and thinking about me and sends her love *(of course that is a given).*

Jim Harras (brother-in-law) wrote at 8:00 AM, figuring it was the moment we were speaking with the docs.

Special entry today from Janie Gordon, my friend who suggested CB to begin with; she wrote, "Hey there my friend! I just finished reading your journal entries and you made me laugh, cry, and shake my head in agreement. You have the right attitude! Keep the faith, stay informed, weigh your options and trudge onward and upward. The cryotherapy sounds awesome. So that would mean no chemo??? I would give anything not to have had to do that. Take it one day at a time, one step in front of the next. So glad you are sleeping better. It took me a long time to sleep through the night. That feeling of "dread" would come over me and I just couldn't stop thinking about the crappy card I had just been dealt. So shocking, so overwhelming, so life changing. But each day gets a little easier and having the positive attitude and spirit is a priceless kind of medicine. Keep it up buddy. You can WHIP this. Love you and Miss you!"

Part of the decision making part of this process is weighing in everyone's opinion. They are all valid opinions. Tim said to "get rid of the sucker." Janie likes the cryotherapy option. Some people rave about U of M, while others rave about Karmanos. I have to put it all in this thing I call my brain and decide on a life-changing event.

Jeannie's two oldest sisters also wrote (Pat and Cathy). Pat wrote that it seemed like a lot to absorb *(DUH)*. She said to keep mulling it over and to remember "<u>Our God is an Awesome God</u>" and to keep asking for guidance. Cathy was sorry that the news was so confusing. She said, "May be no consolation, but it seems that everyone we have known who's been diagnosed with cancer gets the same sort of conflicting messages *(Misery loves company)*. She was amazed how long the tumor was living in my body and is pleased that I am having the other symptoms checked out *(Dr. Hafez didn't give me a choice).*

Saturday, March 5th was a quiet day. I did not write. Just Jim Harras and Aunt May spoke in the CB. Aunt May talked about my need to trust. She quoted the televangelist Joel Osteen who said, "Life is not fair, but know this, God is fair; nothing you have been through has kept you from your destiny. He is in control." *I am always inspired by Joel. I have been to see him live twice and have spent countless hours reading his books and listening to his cds. He is one of the most positive people I know. He has a perpetual smile and any time I am down I can turn to Joel and be uplifted. One of his CDs has a song that says, "I have a friend in God, I have a friend in God, He calls me friend. (I am humming it now). Isn't it unbelievable that as powerful as God is that God can call me his friend? And I truly accept that friendship.*

Another motivational speaker I truly admire is Zig Ziglar. He started life as a salesman, although not a very good one. As his skills improved so did his speaking ability; thus his career in which his ability excels sprung up. One of his principles that I try to follow state: "If you help somebody else get what they want, somebody will help you get what you want." Pretty strong advice. On one of his cds, he tells the story of a follower who complimented Zig and said that whenever he got down he put in one of Zig's tapes and listened and always was felt better. Zig retorted and said, "why not listen to my tapes before you get depressed and perhaps that depression will never set in. Zig ends most of his tapes challenging me and others to follow the principle of his which I stated above and he say: "When you do I will see you not just at the top, I will see you <u>Over the Top</u> (the title of one of his best-selling books).

Jim Harras said: "Just when you think you have it all figured out, God throws you a curve ball! This is what faith is for. Know that whatever plan God has for us, He will only give us what we can handle." *That expression is certainly true, and I have been reminded of it literally thousands of times during my cancer walk. Usually I smile, but on tough days I think, why does God give me so much responsibility?* Jim goes on to say, "I read an article last year that was titled "Man Plans, God smiles." I think of it often when I don't understand why things happen the way they do. Keep the faith and we will keep the prayers going."

Another of the brothers-in-law who was tremendously supportive throughout my journey was Joe "Babe" Bellino. His wife is Peggy who is a regular contributor to CB. Joe prefers to text, a skill

I will never master. Joe is a strong believer in leaving things in God's hands. Do not let any adverse situation or person rent space in your brain – easier said than done, but so true.

Sunday, March 6th:

I wrote: "I was totally not going to write today, but in addition to providing information, this entry has proven to be somewhat therapeutic. About a week before Ryan proposed to Ellen, he met Jeannie and I at the YMCA to speak with us. The only term that came to mind as far as giving him advice was, "SOONER RATHER THAN LATER." What an appropriate phrase to adapt to my life right now. Since the cancer diagnosis on Feb. 16, we have been totally focused on finding the best way to get rid of the cancer. However, after Friday's consultation, my concern is now trying to figure out what is causing the fatigue (slept 11 hours last night) and lack of appetite. And to be honest, I am struggling to be positive today in this journal. Once the day starts moving, I am sure I will do better and move beyond the "stinkin thinkin." It is tough to think about waiting three more weeks and then there will be more waiting for the test results. Nuts! When I started writing, I told myself I would always sound positive, but I am letting myself stray today and being truthful at the same time. Yesterday we sang at church, "Yahweh's Love will last forever!" and I know it will! Sooner rather than later!"

Camille promises to shout to the Lord, "Three weeks is too long" and is inviting others to do the same. And she challenges me to keep writing no matter what my frame of mind is.

Theresa agrees that three weeks is a very long wait. She promises to carry the cross with me during Lent.

Aunt May talked about all of the support that her entire community of sisters is providing. They have a prayer list outside of their chapel, and on many days other sisters have entered my name before she can. She adds: "When we deal with the known, we seem to deal with it better than the unknown."

Fritzi Bohlmann joined the CB train today. She is a dear friend of ours and was in community with Jeannie 35 years ago. She wrote, "After chatting with you tonight, I thought of a great quote of Lena

Horne's: "It's not the load that breaks you down, it's the way you carry it!" Carry it well my friends, carry it well."

Monday, March 7th:

Today was an interesting day filled with lots of unexpected twists and turns. I received a text message from Jeannie at 1:30 (teachers are not allowed to use cell phones either, but have been known to sneak a text message or two). "Jeannie's text said, 'you will hear something by to' – she meant to type tomorrow, but shortened it. I thought she meant 2:00 today. I thought Jeannie was goofy. NEVER MESS WITH JEANNIE. The phone rang ten seconds later and it was U of M. They were calling to schedule the surgery for three days before I was to meet with Dr. Wang. Confused? Me too! I explained that Dr. Hafez said he would not consider surgery until after I was tested by Dr. Wang. The scheduling nurse said she would work on it and get back to me. What did we do before cell phones? She called back in a couple of hours and said that they were able to move up the appointment with Dr. Wang to this Friday (FOUR DAYS away). Then they have scheduled a pre-op meeting the following Wednesday (16th) at 2:00 PM and the surgery itself is set for March 22nd. One minute we seem to be at a standstill and the next is full steam ahead; almost too much for the old Polack to digest all at once. I then slowed down the nurse and reminded her that I hadn't made a final decision between U of M and Karmanos – she replied that I had to hurry up because the surgery was scheduled for two weeks away."

I was thrilled that the process was moving, an entry for the gratitude journal. It is a shame that it is a practice that I do not apply frequently enough. Why is it in times of trouble that we keep asking God for things, but we forget to be grateful? "Shepherd me O God – beyond my wants, beyond my fears…" "Fear no evil for I am at your side." "Your kindness and mercy follow me all the days of my Life…"

Now I have to pray and think and wait anxiously for Jeannie to come home so we can begin to make sense of all of this. I have a spinning head this is happening so fast. I decided to post on CB and wait for Jeannie.

Interesting email exchange with Brother T today. It started

because I shared with TR an email I got from my CPA, Herb. He said that he knows that "God has special plans for you, I am certain." In my expanded family, all relationships have taken on a personal nature; I am in awe. A large number of people (over 20) have sent me Mass intention cards; three different people have sent relics. So amazing, so much support, but I do have my human moments and I do worry. In addition to the cancer worries, I do have the business worries. This is a challenging year for Burger King. Cancer and Burger King–two pretty big issues. TR is always upbeat: "Chuck, you have never let me down. YOU ARE STILL MY HERO and always will be. We just need a little time and you have to listen to the doctors at U of M. You are in good hands. Patience does not run in the Piotrowski household (*I think I have said that before myself, not sure who is quoting whom.*) You will get through this. We are all walking with you. LOVE, Brother T." *One thing for sure, I sure appreciate the frequent use of the word love from everyone. I also really love the bear hugs.*

Seven CB postings today. *I don't know if all of you friends who post realize how uplifting you are. I know that thousands of people are walking with me, but seeing it in black and white is so powerful. I cry daily as I read the postings.*

The first one today was from Sr. Marge Bassett. I am not sure what Sr. Marge's official title is, but in the old days she would have been called Mother Superior. What a fine lady she is, and her community is so lucky to have her leadership. I met her in January while working on a special project. The night that I called Aunt May to tell her of the cancer diagnosis, I called Sr. Marge first. I wanted somebody that lived with my aunt to be aware of my situation in case Aunt May needed somebody to talk to. I actually asked Sr. Marge if she thought I should tell Aunt May myself. She knew Aunt May was a woman of deep faith and that she could handle it. Sr. Marge, in her entry today, blessed Jeannie and I with the gift of hope.

The Jaskulas are praying "with and for us."

Theresa pointed out that the power of prayer is awesome.

Camille wrote that St. Patrick and St. Joseph give me guidance, "as you travel down another path in your journey. Through it all may your joys be like the capital of Ireland ---------- always doubling." *I just now got it!*

Barb Koster wants to make sure that I keep the cell phone charged at all times so that the timely calls and texts keep coming.

Anne Michels sent more xxoo. She, too, is amazed at how rapidly things are moving all of a sudden. She is sure that whatever we decide will be the best decision.

Gwen wrote that she was pleased that I do not have to wait so long. "The tough decisions that lie ahead will be answered through your thoughts, prayers, education, and writings. Pray and think and don't forget to write. The rest of us are here to pray with you and support the decisions you make."

Aunt May wrote: "Praise the Lord! Good news! He is certainly hearing our prayers. Once U of M has your concerns on their table, things begin to move forward. Now prayers for you and Jeannie to make the right decision."

I went to bed early tonight and missed a call from my cousin Mickey. He and his wife, Chris, and his sister, the infamous JoAnne, have been walking with me throughout. I appreciate their calls and concern. JoAnne and I have become closer now as adults than when we were kids – she and her brother and sister-in-law are treasures in my life.

Tuesday, March 8th:

I started writing today and commented that there was nothing to add to my physical condition and probably wouldn't be until the next appointment at U of M. I talked about the anxiety of waiting and reminded everyone that patience is not a Piotrowski virtue, I could say that daily.

I took time today to say thanks to all of the folks who have written on CB, sent emails, or cards, or Mass intentions, or phone calls, and even two people who have sent relics. One of the relics is from Solanus Casey. Sr. Mary Finn pointed out that he still needs one more miracle – this could be it!

"In a situation like this you realize how deep your support system goes, how wide it stretches. So much support from my loving family, especially my brother TR who hates the computer, but reads these postings daily and has posted. Even my nephew's mother-in-law has been very thoughtful. And speaking of nephews and nieces, you are all so precious and your words are very moving to me. The SSJ sisters and even a former sister (Camille) are pounding the heavens. Friends from Cyprian, Pius, OLOW, IHM sisters, Adrian Dominican sisters, friends from the neighborhood (new and old), Burger King, Pat O'Grady's, Camps Ozanam and Stapleton, Sacred Heart Seminary, and several of my brother's friends from Indiana all are very special to me. So many people I volunteer with at Southshore Hospital on Thursdays. I have lost count at how many states have sent wishes, but I know it is in double digits. And if you do not belong to one of those groups, I am sorry for not mentioning it; it is never my intent to exclude anyone. Aunt May is praying furiously and prays to my dear mom, the original Rita. And my cousin, Lynn Marie, has sent cards and assures me that my godfather (George) is up in Heaven and he, too, is speaking to God on my behalf. And then there is Jeannie's Uncle Earl; we sure love him and miss him–between Jeannie and I and Nonnie and Sr. Joy, we have been sending him all kinds of requests. And he works miracles. I am overwhelmed by your kindness, but don't stop!! Sometimes when the "stinkin thinkin" starts to creep in, I will read the cards or the guestbook or turn off all noise and sit quietly (yes I can be quiet), and I know I will make it because of all of you." I have formulated my personal and updated "Litany of Saints;" you have all been promoted. Amen.

 This seems like a good place to talk about the original Jean Byron, my mother-in-law, whom everyone affectionately calls Nonnie. TR has always said that I hit the jackpot with Nonnie and, coming from a gambler, that is the ultimate compliment. She is the kindest lady and is always there for the entire family. And I know she prays for all of us daily. When I had the Whipple surgery seven years ago, she moved in with Jeannie and stayed by her side. When I came home and visited her at her Au Gres cottage, she had a definite routine in mind for me. Sometimes we had different routines in mind and I affectionately called her, "Mean Jean." I love her dearly and could never thank her enough for all of the kindness she has bestowed on me.

 This night I received a call from Mike "Moose" Morris. He is another seminary buddy who has bonded with me for life. I could share many past memories of things we have done together, it would be enough material for another book. Let me just say that Mike (and now Cathy) are always there for anyone who needs them. Thanks, Guys.

My niece and nephew (Mike and Shannon Pio) sent entries today. They both used the term that they were thinking of me. It's nice to be thought of by a younger generation and even nicer when they both, in two different entries, took time out of their lives to write.

The Jaskulas are always ready to add a little humor, which is certainly a welcome diversion these days. They said, "If we had known you would appreciate relics, we would have stopped over." Hmmm.

Aunt May continues to walk with us. She writes, "It is great hearing from you daily. You have no idea how often your messages are checked so keep it up. It helps your spirits, but ours as well."

Jim and Cheryl Littlepage are great friends from St. Cyprian days; they have been walking with us for 28 years. "You are now officially added to my list of people that I am praying for. May God continue to give you strength on this journey, and guide your physicians in your care." One can never pray enough for the doctors.

Chapter Six

The Verdict Is In!
Week 4

___

Wednesday, March 9th: *4:10 a.m.*

Hard to believe how early these postings can be. If I can't sleep I take advantage of the therapeutic value of writing these entries. My entire entry for this day reads: "One thing that has truly amazed me through this whole process is the availability of the doctors. They truly care. Of course, Rick Klapchar really got the ball rolling and moved things very quickly. At both U of M and Karmanos, I was originally seen by the head nurse (for about an hour) and then the doctor himself spent an additional hour. It is very satisfying to know that I am not a number, but truly a patient and a human being that they care about and want to help. I do want to single out Dr. Ed Nazareno. He is our family doctor, although in modern lingo they call him, "primary care physician." He is truly walking with us. He was the one who gave me the diagnosis of cancer. He was the one we turned to for advice when U of M and Karmanos each strongly suggested radically different paths of treatment. He is younger and readily admitted that he did not have a lot of knowledge of cryotherapy and kidney cancer in general. He said he would do his research and he has! He called yesterday just to talk, not the first time he has done this. He is of the strong opinion, after doing research and talking to his experts, that surgery is the only option to take. He recommends following the path of either laparoscopic or robotic as the best way to go. Due to my health history, Dr. Hafez (U of M) will follow the safest routine possible. THE DECISION IS FINAL! It's off to U of M for sure. Thanks to Rick and Dr. Littrup for presenting another viable option. I know I am in capable hands with Dr. Hafez."

CB writing #1, Aunt May: "I am pleased with your final decision with U of M only because: 1) your health condition has not been the greatest and 2) they asked for more tests before they moved forward, plus they will follow up after surgery. God is good having you at peace with your decision. I'm with you all the way so is your dear Mom. I, too, have been praying to her for guidance."

CB writing #2, Camille: "I'd say you have made a wise decision. The angel of the sick is Rapheal. The Archangel, called the medicine of God, drives away diseases of the body and brings health to our minds (from a hymn in the Divine Office). He is the physician in care of our health, may he come to care for all who are sick. Now we ask the Angel Rapheal to guide your physicians, to enlighten and bless them as they treat you. Breathe easy today!"

CB #3, My niece Amy (from Wisconsin–another state heard from): "So glad you've made your decision! We will continue to pray for you!!"

CB #4, Theresa: "May peace continue to fill you. Prayers."

CB #5, Pat and Bruce: "So happy that you have been able to make the decision on what path to follow. It has got to be one huge relief for you. Your confidence in your decisions helps all of us more forward! We continue to pray for restored health for you."

CB #6, The Jaskulas (the relics): "Boy…I can feel the peace with which you have come to your decision to have surgery. If you go into the surgery with that same sense of peace and confidence… you will come out of it the same way."

Thursday, March 10th I wrote: "About a week ago somebody asked me what my favorite word was. Instantly and without hesitation I said, "BUS!" He was amazed and wanted to know why. I reminded him that I own a fast food restaurant and a BUS mean lots of instant business. Tomorrow's appointment at U of M is not until 9:30 AM so I will drop a note subsequent to that visit. Hope you all have plenty of your versions of "BUSSES" in your lives today."

CB #1, Cousin Mickey and Chris: "We were at church last night. We lit a candle for you AND for your doctor. We want you to get well and your doctor to do everything right. Good Luck!"

CB #2, Sr. Marge: "Continuing to pray for both of you. I will pray also for the doctors as you prepare for this next step in the journey. May God grant wisdom to these skilled physicians and surgeons as they journey with you."

CB #3 and 4, Camille: "When I left for Mass this morning, we were engulfed in a blanket of fog. When I left the church (out the front door) the Lake was suddenly visible, like an instant happening. May your future appointments hold no fogs for you, just instant (BUS) results. Hope you can enjoy this day as your prepare for Friday's tests! I forgot to say that I attend Mass as St. Paul's on the Lake. It is a beautiful vista any time of the day, but mornings are special."

CB#5, Aunt May wished me good luck tomorrow and safe travelling.

Thought for the day: "Unforgiveness is like cancer; it will eat you from the inside out." Start forgiving!

Friday, March 11th I wrote: "Long day today (*The entry was not posted until 7:41 PM, most days I have the entry done before 6:00 AM*). Why does it always seem to snow when we have an appointment at U of M? First meeting today was with Dr. Wang (gastro guy) to determine if there were any other reasons as to the weight loss and fatigue. I did not know what to expect and was prepared for a barrage of tests, not the case. Dr. Wang entered the room and towered over us. We had a nice long talk. Reason #1 is obviously the cancer. Reason #2 is that I take enzymes with every meal to artificially do the work of my missing pancreas. Dr. Wang feels that I only take half the dose of what I need. What a relief; it is a quick and easy fix and so now I have switched brands and take twice the amount of pills.

Then we met with the scheduling nurse. We are still on for the 22nd, but she does not have a clue as to the time. Dr. Hafez does two surgeries a day (AM and PM). And the calendar is not set for that day. They have also not decided as to whether or not it will be open surgery or robotic surgery. There are twelve docs on the team and the nurse says that my case gets emailed about daily (*would be interesting to read those dialogues*) discussing the pros and cons of both methods; no decisions made yet and will probably not be made until a day or two before the surgery. We are MOVING FORWARD.

REALITY CHECK #1:

Putting things in perspective; we took Matt and Rob to a high school basketball game at Detroit County Day. One of their coaches is a friend from high school whom I haven't seen in years. He looked at me, put his arm around me, and said he wasn't doing too well. He is in the process of getting a divorce after 35 years of marriage. All of a sudden it made my kidney cancer look like a bee sting. My prayer tonight is for that coach and his struggle in life. (*Sadly the divorce decree was final the day of my surgery.*)

Mike and Linda Meyers (another High School chum) wrote: "Thinking about you and just wanted you to know that we will be with you every step of the way in our hearts, thoughts, and of course our prayers."

Aunt May wrote: "Thanks for your call from the U of M parking lot. I am thankful that all went well for you and hopefully they know what they should do about the weight loss. I felt your report was great and now we move forward to the pre-op and then the surgery. How are you holding up Jeannie? Thanks for your support and loving care for Chuck." *The best way that I can answer that question is to say that Jeannie is amazing. Throughout this whole ordeal she has been upbeat and positive. There is no doubt that surgery will be successful. I know that part of the time she is down she turns to the Lord. I am not sure where else she goes when she has her "down time." I know the Lord is smiling on her and saying, "Well done good and faithful servant."*

From a random Internet motivational source: "Every day you are getting closer. Everything you have ever wanted is being pressed toward you. Everything is clicking. Don't let the illusions trick you. Don't let the events of today dampen your spirits. Things couldn't be any better than they are now. You couldn't have any more reason to celebrate. Now! Do it! The hardest work is done! Just show up, be present, open every door and let events unfold. Life is your stage. This is your parade. Together we can do anything. Amen.

Thought for the day: "The reason for all challenges is so that you can finally learn that none are bigger than you." Amen

My writing on Saturday, March 12th: "Great night's sleep with yesterday's appointment out of the way. I do not always admit to the amount of anxiety I have. I just got done finishing a U of M survey. I am being asked to fill out a weekly survey describing how I feel, and how I feel about how I feel. I HAVE NOT met a doc or a nurse who didn't care and who ever made me feel rushed.

REALITY CHECK #2:

At the game yesterday I heard a heartbreaking story. A basketball player from another school is a 17 year old German exchange student. Two weeks ago he got arrested with the charge of "Minor in Possession." He called his parents in Germany several times to explain and to apologize. They were not very understanding and he became very frustrated with each rejection. He saw only one solution; he jumped off a six story building to an instant death. How forgiving and understanding am I? Do I take time to listen to my kids or to anyone who exhibits a need? Once again this story makes my cancer seem like a minor cough. Please pray for that kid and his family."

Camille wrote: "Happy to hear your test went well. They do produce a ton of anxiety. Reading about the young man who died, it made me reflect on the students who I have lost over the years. The pain their parents experienced is still with them today. Enjoy this Saturday and I hope you see or hear from YOUR children today. *Of course, one of my children lives with me. His sister lives minutes away, but I hear from her daily. Her brother lives half a country away, but during this cancer walk he too, calls daily. I felt the pain of the exchange student's parents; glad I hug mine daily!!*

Theresa congratulated me on the weight loss and is praying for a smooth and quick recovery.

Sunday, March 13th:

Jeannie wrote today: "Nothing really new to report today. Charlie has been pretty tried. He tries to rest and cannot; tries to read and cannot concentrate. He can't even enjoy MATLOCK, one of his favorite TV shows. A week from Tuesday cannot get here soon enough. We so appreciate all the love and prayerful support."

Aunt May wrote, "Good hearing from you Jeannie. This time must be most difficult for all of you. I know I find the waiting difficult, also. Just want to make sure that Ellen will be with you at the time of surgery. I will be there in spirit and in prayer. *A day or two later Aunt May sent one of her many greeting cards, telling us that she would be happy to be with us at U of M on the day of surgery. We thanked her for her offer, but knew that there were at least three people who would be with Jeannie, no need to inconvenience her.*

The Kulis wrote to Jeannie to thank her for the updates and to remind us that. "He is in our prayers."

Peg and Joe said: "Thanks for the updates Pios! Full speed ahead and, as always, you have all our prayers!"

Monday, March 14th:

"I was sitting at my desk at Burger King, catching up on some paper work when my cell phone rang. Instantly I looked at Caller ID (can one answer the phone without sneaking a peak) and realized that it was U of M calling. "Now what?" I exclaimed. It seems that my docs have been reviewing my CT scan and have decided they would like to do a bone scan before the surgery. My family doc did tell me a month ago that there were some irregularities with my lower spine. All of that did take a back seat to the cancer diagnosis. So now Dr. Hafez wants to do a bone scan. It will be Wednesday. I now have five different U of M appointments all scheduled for Wednesday; two dealing with the bone scan and three others dealing with pre-op stuff. The scheduling nurse today was very reassuring when she commented that it is always better to have as much information as is available before doing surgery. So Wednesday will be another test. Wednesday will also be one month exactly since I was told I have cancer. Holding all of you so close."

There were nine responses to this entry. Even as I reread them now, I continue to get so much support from everybody every day. And so many people communicate in other forms than CB. I talk to TR several times each day. Sprint loves us. I am amazed and humbled by the volumes of care and concern I feel. And I know that, as I proceed in life, I will try to pass out the love to others in need more freely. Once again, interesting to note that four of the comments are coming from SSJs; what a prayerful and supporting group of women these ladies are. Should you ever have an intention, get on their prayer list and it will soon be "Mission Accomplished."

As always, Aunt May was the first to respond. I sometimes wonder if she stays in the computer lab waiting for my entries. "Well, again it looks like U of M continues to study your case making sure they have all of the facts. This pleases me that they are on top of your case. Wednesday is not that far away."

Theresa says, "It's nice that they want the best for you! Prayers for a quick recovery."

Camille made me smile when she said: "Do you remember the song – "My mama told me there would be days like this?" Hang in there and cross the days off. Put a favorite medal or rosary in your pocket and when you can't get it together, just squeeze that the best you can. Prayers for the Family." *Interesting thing is that for several years now I always carry two such items in my pocket. One is a sterling silver cross with the Serenity Prayer on the cross. The other is a bead that was given to me by my son, Joe, when he was going through some tough times. He asked me to always carry it and say a prayer for him anytime I felt the bead in my pocket. Several rosaries later……..*

Sr. Marge wrote: "Continuing to pray for you daily. May God be with you as you continue to undergo tests and preparation for surgery. May God inspire each of the doctors with whom you are working. You are both an inspiration. Your faith and trust are shining examples. Thank you for sharing your story. *Once again I digress to say that I continue to feel like I have just taken another slice of humble pie. In the short time I have gotten to know Sr. Marge, I am amazed at her keen sense of togetherness. This is true in the case of her leadership of the community. It is also true in the case of bonding with me, one of her newest friends. She is an incredible lady!*

Mike and Linda comment on how busy Wednesday will be. They told me to relax. LOL. They added, "You will be in very good hands and we pray that God will give the Doc and Techs all the knowledge, compassion, and dedication to help all of you through this." Then they bragged about the beautiful day up north (they live in Indian River), thankfully they were willing to share the day.

Janie, my cancer survivor buddy wrote: "Well my friends…

welcome to the world of hospitals, tests and more tests. Even though it may sound never-ending *(that is an under-statement)*, it is well worth it in the long run. It sounds like your docs are very thorough and that is the most reassuring thing when you feel like you have lost control of so much. The waiting is also hard when you are expecting answers. Chuck... just know that so many are praying for you and for your doctors. You are never alone. The footprints poem helped me through times. I would read it over and over to remind me that it was ok to let go and let God. Having one set of footprints in the sand is such a gentle and gracious reminder of how much we are loved and cared for by our Lord and Savior. Blessings to you both and keep the faith my friend. YOU CAN DO THIS!" And she ends with xxoo and much love.

Barb Koster points out that it is great that people are reading and reviewing and thinking over my case as I am waiting for the next appointment. She said that I am in good hands – and her prayer is that God will guide all of those talented hands and minds.

Anne Michels reminded me that it was the old Daylight savings time switch this weekend which makes for a tiring and trying weekend. She thanked me for the posts and updates.

Another great thing that Ann Marie did was to let her brother and sister-in-law know of my situation. I worked with both Sheri and Rick at Pat O'Gradys in the mid 70's. I have not seen or heard from them is thirty years, as they now live in California. They wrote: "Chuck it's been too long. Just heard about what is going on and want you to know that you will be in our prayers daily. We want you to know that, "God is the God of all comfort, and He will comfort you so that you may comfort others." God Bless you and we love you."

Tuesday, March 15th:

"Good day to one and all – "I am surrounded by God's grace and surrounded by people filled with God's grace!" This is my new mantra and will be repeated by me several times in the next seven days, months, years, etc. Jeannie's comment on Sunday talked about my anxiety–gosh was I a mess (that's why I didn't even write). I was very weak and allowed some depression to set in. I would read some of your comments and you would talk about our faith and I would think to myself: "They wouldn't be saying that if they knew where I was at this weekend." Jeannie and I have a wonderful partnership. Unfortunately, I have not been the best partner this last month. She is getting the raw end of the deal. She is always strong and supportive, never asking for anything in return. She sure picked up the slack, of course she has been doing that for years–even when I once introduced her as Jackie *(and just the other day I called her Ellen, at least I can explain Ellen, never have figure out where Jackie came from.)* So yesterday I made some time for a mid-course correction and **I feel awesome today. You should see me smiling!!** When I feel anxious I will take a deep breath in and suck in all of God's grace *(well I guess I can save some for you.)* When I exhale I will blow out all of that stupid anxiety (which is put there by the devil.). Each day I am more comfortable with the decision to go to U of M. I am glad for the extra test tomorrow, which will only make the doc's decision about the type of surgery I need to have easier to discern. Hope you have an awesome day today–I sure plan to!"

The Chirco family responded by saying, "Wow! We can sure see your smile this morning! Please keep the faith as everyone has been telling you these past few weeks and days. God will get you, Jeannie, and the rest of the family through this difficult time. We will think of you tomorrow and every day until this is all over."

Aunt May wrote, "Isn't the saying behind every good man there is a good woman? Well Jeannie has proven this to be so true. You are doing great, Chuck. Yes, you will have days that will get you down; but, once again, your faith and trust will spring you back to your feet; "all will be well."

Kris Jaskula wrote, "I am surrounded by God's grace and by people filled with God's grace… that is truly an amazing mantra. With all humility may I offer an even easier one…? JESUS… say it over and over and over again. In the book <u>The Wonders of the Holy Name</u>, we learn that Jesus is an all-powerful prayer and that whatever we ask the Father in His name we shall receive. It goes on to say that each time we say the name "Jesus" it is an offering of perfect love; it saves us from the power of the devil, who is always ready to do us harm (in thoughts and deeds), it fills us with peace and joy and it gives us strength to bear our sufferings. Every time I think of you and Jeannie, I pray…

"Jesus, Jesus, Jesus" and offer up any graces I may receive to you. God bless… keep smiling… and know He is with you."

Anne Stehle wrote: "Good day to both you and Jeannie. Chuck, you gave me strength this morning when I read your thoughts about anxiety. I will remember to breathe in all of God's goodness and breathe out the anxiety. My worries are small, but nonetheless, they get to me. This moving business has tired me out and it makes it hard to deal with the stressors in my life. Mom turns 90 today. You are in my daily thoughts and prayers. Blessings do come from tragedy. I have been blessed with more contact with you and Jeannie and getting to know the most beautiful inner you." *(Thanks for all of the kind words Anne, I have probably read this passage half a dozen times, but reading it today continues to move me. I never think of myself as having a "beautiful inner you," so I thank Anne for recognizing that in me. In addition to what Anne has written here, she has sent many emails and has friends in high places at U of M and she has gotten answers to many questions for me.)*

Cheryl Littlepage is still hugging me, thank God. She continues: "to pray for your doctors' intelligence in the correct way to treat you. And I continue to pray that you will get through this difficult trial, healthy. I would have to say, however, it seems as if it is you who seems to be lifting US up with all your good will. I am not sure that I could be that positive; I pray that I would be. Continue to stay focused on your faith road, and I will continue to pray for you."

Theresa reminds me that we all have days in which we need someone to pick up the slack. Honesty and faith will keep you moving forward.

Joy Baker is a Sylvanian Franciscan sister who was close friends with Uncle Earl. She has subsequently become a close friend of ours. She writes: "You have full support in this time of waiting. I truly hold you in prayer and ask God to hold you and your concerns/family in his loving arms! God can do far more that I could ever hope for you!"

All contact is greatly appreciated more than anyone probably realizes. The fact that people have chosen to stay in contact with me through daily readings of CB and the many who respond with comments is mind blowing. As of today (July 1st) there have been 2972 comments posted on CB – WOW! Plus every now and then somebody will call or email and say they read the journal daily, but chose not to write. It is just warming to know that they care. Never any doubt that folks care, but the message sure has come through, big time.

One of the most amazing comments I received today came in the form of an email from Barb Koster. She writes: Chuck didn't both your parents donate their bodies to U of M for research? It's probably not possible to know how your parents contributed to the science of medicine, but I want to believe that what researchers learned from your parents will be used to chase your cancer! Thanks to Hank and Rita for yet more gifts!! The amazing circle of life." *Barb is 100% correct. Both of my parents did indeed donate their bodies to U of M for research. They used Hank's remains for several months and then he was cremated. In June of the following year, a most amazing memorial service was held for the families of all the faithful who had donated their bodies. The service was held at Washtenog Ceremony is Whitmore Lake (home of our Burger King). Hundreds of folks were present. Rita and I went and represented our family. A string quartet played music in the background. A small portion of their glee club was present to provide comforting music. The chaplain offered an invocation. The highlight of the day was four speeches from different interns. I clearly remember the first speech fifteen years later. The young doctor (looked younger than my kids) gave an emotional tribute to Hank and all of the others. He called the class of '97 his first "real teacher." There is information to be obtained from the lectures and text books. Nothing is more significant than "hands-on" experience. He quietly sobbed as he spoke and could not thank the families enough for the generous donations of the remains of their loved ones. There was not a dry eye in the house – I, in fact, am quietly crying now as I write this. Rita's homecoming came in 2004. Once again, when U of M had finished using her remains, we were contacted and invited to a similar memorial service. TR, Patsy, and I attended this time. It was so special to be there with my two siblings. The service was pretty much the same. This time in the front of the tent there was a huge coffin that housed the cremains of those kind donors. It was a stark reality to see that flag-draped coffin. Proud to say that, twenty years ago, Jeannie and I made arrangements to donate our bodies to Wayne State. At the time U of M was not accepting bodies. We figured helping future doctors and nurses at Wayne State was equally as important. Thanks Barb, you made a moving, emotional, and satisfying observation. Who knows specifically what Hank and Rita were able to do for my situation. I certainly know that the knowledge the doctors obtained from my parents definitely did help my case.*

My Childhood

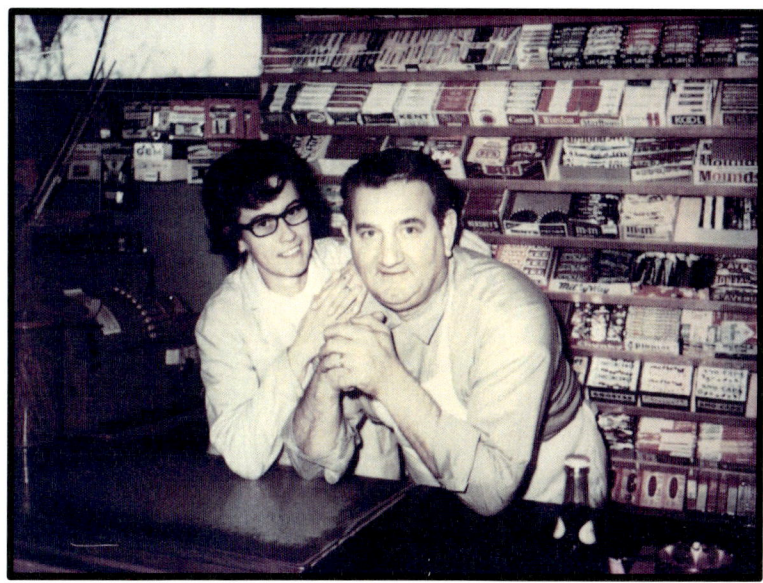

My parents, Hank and Rita, at Handee Food Centre
1972

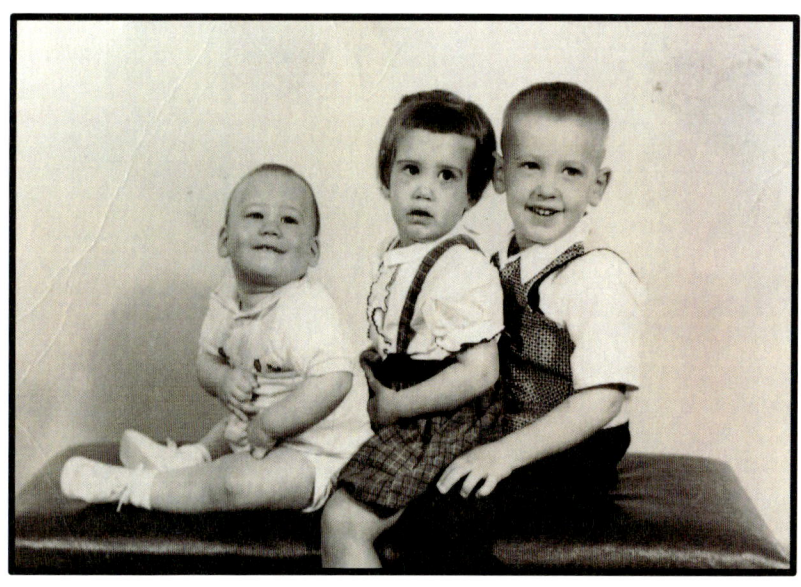

Piotrowski kids growing up
1954

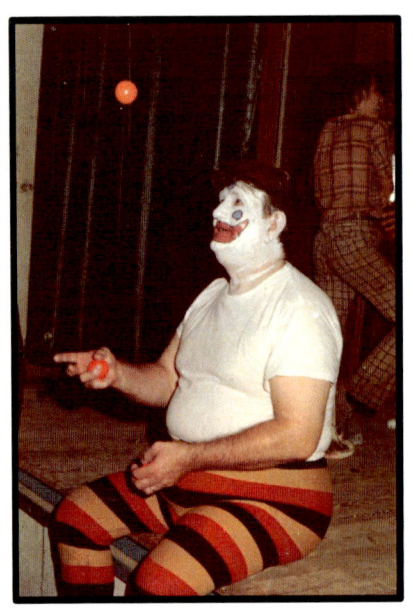

Hanko the Clown,
Chuck's dad at Camp Ozanam
1975

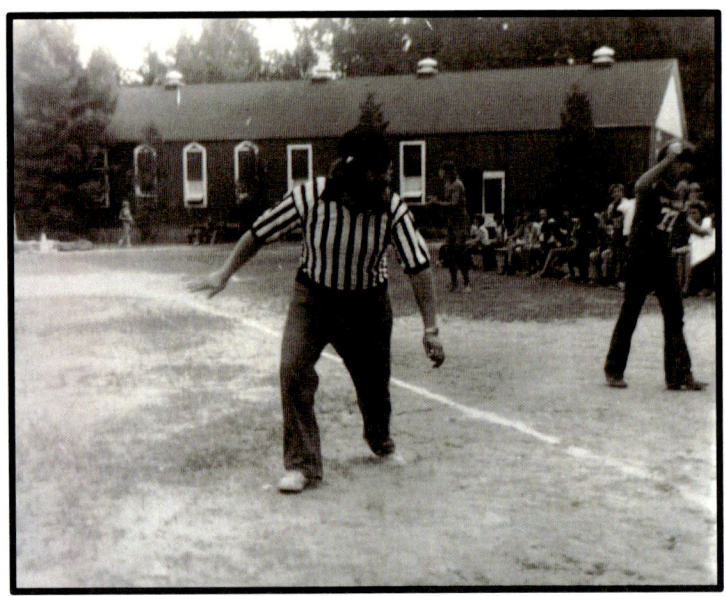

Chuck umpiring a baseball game at Camp Ozanam
1974

Chapter Seven

The Final Countdown
Week 5

Thought for the day: "You can't let tough stuff get in the way of moving forward." Moving forward is the key.

Wednesday, March 16th:

What a day!

7:00 AM:

We checked in for the Bone scan. I had to be injected with some kind of dye that will help the technicians read the test. Being injected only took a matter of minutes. Because it was a new area of U of M, we had to give all of my information again. Once the dye was injected we had several hours to kill.

8:00 AM:

We walked to a near restaurant that is a local favorite, Angelo's. It came highly recommended by my godson, Patrick Meyers. He highly recommended their home-made French toast. Being an expert of fine foods, we knew Pat would not let us down. The meal was outstanding, but way too much food.

9:00 AM:

We walked back to U of M and had to wait for two more hours. Believe it or not, we had to fill out my medical history again.

11:00 AM:

Time for the bone scan. Once again I was placed on a platform and rolled into a machine. I had to lie perfectly still for several seconds (seemed like minutes) while the machine took the pictures. It turned out that two of the pictures did not take so I had to have two retakes (sounds like school pictures). Results are not immediately available, but they are, just not to me. Now we had two hours to kill before our next appointment.

1:00 p.m.:

This appointment was on the other side of US 23 at Domino Farms; U of M has run out of room in the main hospital. Our appointment was with Dr. Jimbo in the Department of Japanese medicine. I was sure we were in the wrong place. Even the graphics on the door were in Japanese, but the number was what it said on my schedule sheet, so we went in. First order of business was to fill out my medical records (surprise!). The purpose of this visit was for this doctor to give his approval as to my readiness for surgery. He was very thorough in his questions. He had an intern with him, who smiled and nodded. They told me I was done and they would give their findings to Dr. Hafez.

2:30 PM:

We had to drive to a different part of Domino Farms for more tests. You guessed it; I had to fill out my medical history for the fourth time today. Maybe they act as lie detector tests to see if I answer the same every time. A familiar-looking girl was taking my vital signs. I glanced at her name tag and said, "Sarah, do you remember me, you used to work for me at Burger King." Sure enough about seven years earlier she worked for me. Isn't it amazing how small the world is? Sarah passed me off to another lady, who took blood and did more records. I asked the second lady if she could tell, by reading my records, what type of surgery they were planning. She turned on the computer and informed me that at that moment the verdict was to do the surgery robotically. That pleased me because the surgery is less invasive and the recovery faster. They did warn me that once the surgery began, there is a chance they may have to switch to open surgery to avoid any complications. No clue as to the time of surgery.

All I knew was that I was tired and I didn't do anything. Time to go home and unwind. It just amazes me how little energy I have. The first thing I did when I got home was to check email. I received an amazing email from one of my nephews, Chris Bernhold. Chris lives in Phoenix and we do not have much contact. He is a great kid and I know he is always there. He wrote: "Hi Uncle Pio and Aunt Jeannie. A book I read years ago had a line: "Words bend emotions, like sticks in water," and it's in times like these that it resonates. Since Uncle Pio has been thrown this curveball there has not been a day that goes by that the both of you, Joey, Ellen, and Matt have not been in my heart, thoughts, and prayers. You may have heard this line before, I don't know who authored it: "Don't tell God how big your storm is; tell the storm how big your God is!" Over the last couple of years I have drawn great strength from it and hope, in sharing it with you both, it can help you in this trying time. And he signed Love Always, Christopher."

*Love is something that is always understood and too often taken for granted. As Chris wrote those words it moved me as so many others before have moved me. We don't express love enough. My challenge to all of you reading this book **right now** is to put the book down and call somebody that is special to you and tell them you love them. For me, I am stopping for the night, but I plan to email Chris right now and tell him I love him. Isn't love grand? Think of waiting up for your kid to come home at 1:30 AM from washing dishes – that is true love!*

Five CB entries today. As usual, my morning prayer and good wish come from Aunt May. Cheryl Littlepage is a great hugger as all of her entries end with more hugs. She was quite moved by my nephew's quote, telling the storm how big my God is. Aunt May also got (?) on a second time, twelve hours later. She commented, in response to Barb Koster's email, that my mom and dad are with me as I move forward. John and Ruth Maxwell (their son is married to my niece–we are all one big family) are keeping us in their thoughts and prayers. They are keeping positive thoughts! John commented: "Keep up the fight brother, you can beat this!"

Camille wrote: "Prayed to your guardian angel *(glad they have not been retired)* that he would be with you each step of the way. Tomorrow we shall celebrate the Irish. My wish is that the Luck of the Irish be with you and may four leaf clovers be on your path." She said that she would mention my struggle to her pastor, Pat Halfpenny, who was a few years ahead of me in the seminary. She concluded, "May God Bless – it has been a long day for the ENTIRE family." *Family is not just the five Piotrowskis, but also everyone who is walking with me. I have a BIG family.*

On Thursday, March 17th, there was not much new for me to share. We are all Irish today. My mom was so proud of her heritage. Every year since her death I get a call from my cousin, Joanne. Even she (who is Polish/Hungarian) is Irish today. I did mention in my posting that after Mass on Sunday, Rick Macey would be giving me The Sacrament of the Sick and I invited anyone to come. I concluded with my mantra: "We are surrounded by God's grace and with people who are filled with God's grace."

Aunt May was happy to hear that I would be anointed. She assures me all will be well. Her close friend, Theresa, thanked me for my deep faith! *Comments like Theresa's are always very humbling. I don't view my faith as that deep as I have many questions and weak moments. I do know that my faith does grow stronger daily because of my Family.*

Friday, March 18 I wrote: "Spring is here and boy am I ready to celebrate this spring more than ever. I forgot to relay a significant detail from Wednesday at U of M. I was being tested in one of their clinics and the nurse was asking a bunch of questions. She clicked on the computer screen to get info and all at once she looked at me and smiled. I asked her what that was all about. She had just come to know that Dr. Hafez was my surgeon. She exclaimed, 'I just love Dr. Hafez! He is the best surgeon that U of M has!' What an awesome unsolicited testimonial! Very comforting to know that I have the best!"

"Also on Wednesday, Ellen attended the funeral of Fr. Wytral, retired pastor of St. Stephen's. If you know Ellen, she sticks to her comfort zone and doesn't do much mingling. But she saw a priest that she thought she recognized. She approached him (probably nervously) and confirmed her suspicions – she was with Fr. Prus. He is truly one of the Spiritual Giants in my life. Ellen told Fr. Prus of my kidney cancer diagnosis and he assured her of his prayer for me. It was instantly uplifting to know that I was included in Fr. Prus's prayer list. But he did one better – he called yesterday – we had a delightful chat and then we prayed together over the phone. And he promised to keep including me in his daily rosaries. Does it get any better than that? Thanks again for all of your support as well. Each day I continue to be humbled because of all you kindnesses and prayers. The beast is beaten and almost removed!"

Brother T wrote today: "Cancer SUCKS. Thank God next Tuesday it will be out! Focus on your faith, let God deal with the rest. You are a great brother (MY HERO). We will do anything for each other. We are there for you. All will be just FINE."

Cathy (sister-in-law) said that my daily notes are inspirational. *Hmm, humbled again.*

Sr. Marge wrote: "God is awesome in the way that he knows what we need. I am so pleased that you continue to find encouragement and solace in the people and events around you. Such a positive attitude is so helpful in the healing process. May God continue to send you uplifting signs that He is with you and holding you in His heart."

Linda Meyers wrote that I sounded good *(and she is right I was feeling good).* She enjoyed the story about my mom and dad donating their bodies to the U of M. She pointed out that her dad also donated lots of samples and tissues in 2007 at U of M. She is proud of his cooperation with their research and now it seems as if he is helping someone very special to her.

Cousin, Joannie, said: "Good to hear your positive attitude when talking today, keep that up. These little twist and turns we go through just make us stronger. I'm sure that with all of us praying for you, the Lord will get the message loud and clear. Put it in His hands."

Jim Vedro (friend) is as computer-challenged as I am. He finally got some help in figuring out how to enter this website. Jim has been calling every few days, sharing his wisdom and support. Thank you Jim for always being there, from beautiful Minnesota.

Saturday, March 19th:

This entry was written at 3:03 AM. Guess I couldn't sleep that night. "Day 31 of living with cancer. Good Morning – Today will be another amazing day in this wonderful journey of life. Last night Jeannie and I went to visit a neighbor, who just discovered that he has prostate cancer. He is devastated. He doesn't know where to turn. He is saying: "Why me" (sound familiar?) He has only known about his cancer for seven days and I have 31 days under my belt – it makes me the expert! This man is a customer on Matt's route and often seems to find something wrong. But he is one of God's chosen and we went to visit hoping to be able to help him out and we left his house knowing that we did. The greatest strength that I have is the faith that God has blessed me with, which is supported by all of you. My faith is the biggest asset in my bag of tricks. Hopefully he can reach in his bag of tricks and have the same results. Things are tough for him right now. Somebody gave him the idea that he is going to have to live in diapers the rest of his life. I told him that ain't happening with me and I KNOW that it ain't gonna happen for him either. We assured him that we are walking down the road with him and we will conquer the beast together. *Sad to say that we are not too close with him, but as of today (July 4th) he has not had any treatment. We understand he has done lots of research, but has not been able to reach a decision that he could be comfortable with. Thank God I was able to reach a quick and proper decision.* During Holy Week there is a Litany of Saints that we use at our parish and part of the refrain is, "All you holy men and women pray for us." YOU ARE MY HOLY MEN AND WOMEN. You lift me up in prayer and Tuesday when I will be laying on that operating table getting ready for surgery, I will be singing that refrain praying for all of you who mean so much to me. Can you see me smiling now? Good thing you can't hear my singing, as that is not one of my strengths.

Mary Kuli wrote on CB that she enjoyed seeing the photo that was put up on our website. She pointed out that her husband, whom our kids affectionately call "Dickie-Doo," went through prostate cancer in 2009 and he got through it fairly well by going through radiation.

Theresa said: "Keep singing; your attitude and prayers will destroy the beast! Prayers!"

The Jaskulas wrote: "God bless you all!! We will be with you in spirit on Tuesday."

Camille wrote about Msgr. Canfield (former rector of SHS). He has asked her: "What was the highlight of your journey?" She enjoyed the highlights from my journal as expressed above. And appropriately wished me a Happy St. Joseph Day.

Sheri and Rick wrote again from California: "God is already using you to be a comfort to others."

Aunt May complimented me when she said, "Reaching out to others has always been one of your gifts. No wonder so many have taken the time to reach out to you. You are doing great and the Lord continues to bless you for the many lives you have touched."

Sunday, March 20th was a busy day. I started by thanking Ellen for posting our picture on CB. Of course, she used a picture from her wedding: which was truly a perfect day. We are one proud family. Church today was awesome. Fr. Rick invited all of us around the font for the anointing. All of those friends present were invited to place their hand on me as he prayed; so powerful and uplifting. In his homily today, Fr. Rick talked about one of his personal favorite phrases to meditate on, "how good it is to be here in this place." I knew how good it was for me to be anointed with all who are walking with me, whether they were at church or there in spirit. And I know I will be meditating on this thought on Tuesday before and after surgery. At the anointing somebody said that they would be praying for me. I reminded them that it is important to pray for Dr. Hafez too. TR and his family are on vacation. I told him that I would soon be going on an all-inclusive trip as well – to Ann Arbor – which includes all drinks and meals, too.

Jeannie and Ellen were off to one of their shopping trips to Target. What is so special about that store? How much can one buy there? But most Sundays they go there and Ellen is emphatic that I not go along. So I stayed home and rested. Mike Morris called. Jay Yule called. Thanks for great friends. I did a lot of pacing. Then the phone rang again and I immediately checked caller id (we've talked about this before). I did not recognize the number so I answered. Imagine my surprise and pleasure when I learned it was Dr. Hafez himself, calling a patient on a Sunday afternoon. It is quite a testimony as to the character of this gentleman who will be performing my surgery. I retold the story from church this morning when I asked my friend to pray for Dr. Hafez. He paused for a second and then said, "God Bless

You!" That was powerful the doctor asking God to bless me. Dr. Hafez was very upbeat; he said that all of the testing from the last two weeks has been extremely positive. He is not worried about the surgery, but has changed his mind and feels that the best form of surgery would be open surgery. This contradicts the decision from three days ago, but I am perfectly fine with open surgery; it means longer surgery and longer recovery, but he feels it is the most effective way to go. He will continue to monitor me every three months for the next couple of years, but his feeling is that once he removes the cancer, I am "good to go for another 30 years!" That would give me a life span of 89!! *A little trivia here: My mom, dad, and godfather all died when they were 78. I have since determined that I will never see 78 – I plan to go from 77 directly to 79 – and will now keep counting until 89!* He said my diabetes and the fact that my pancreas has shriveled up (due to earlier surgery) are his two biggest concerns. So if I faithfully take my pancreas enzyme pills (Yes, Jeannie, I promise) and monitor my weight I should be good to go. So incredible, I am praying for Dr. Hafez and he is praying for me. I am in awe that he called and spent half an hour with me on a Sunday afternoon. He is pretty sure that the surgery will be in the afternoon on Tuesday, as he has a major case in the morning. I was glad for that because Matt is winning some kind of Academic Award in the morning and I would like to be there for that presentation. Dr. Hafez said, "That settles it – the surgery will definitely be in the afternoon – go see your kid." How considerate.

    We decided to make Sunday supper simple. We invited over the Baginskis and the Simons. We bowl with them every Sunday night; this would be my final time bowling. I have been known to jump on the lanes to try and knock down that extra pin. I am the anchor of the team. I sink or should I say stink. Truth of the matter is, since I was not able to complete the season they had to use my current average. Sad to say it was only 89 – so that low average allowed our team to coast for a first place finish in the El Cheapo league. The supper was special, being with family and friends and enjoying one of my all-time favorites–Sloppy Joes. The meeting was topped off by my favorite dessert, lemon meringue pie, supplied by my buddy, Elaine Simon. Tomorrow is a day of a complete liquid diet. Followed by a cleansing–Yuk!

As you can imagine, quite a few comments on CB:

Kris Jaskula wrote, "Chuck and Dr. Hafez seem to be a perfect fit…you two were undoubtedly meant to cross paths…even if it is for this little detour in life… God Bless you both."

Anne Marie Michel complimented our picture. I haven't seen Anne in over ten years. She said the picture was a "beautiful sight of love." We appreciate, resemble, and accept that compliment.

Joy was also amazed that the doctor took the time to call on a Sunday. "The doctor is praying for you as you pray for him and we all pray for you and your family – what a chain of prayer!"

Joanne Schiegelone saw Matt at a play last night and asked him to relay a message, which she was afraid he would forget (she was right). She wished me "the best on Tuesday. It is the beginning of the road to beat the Big C. I sure do know what you are going through all too well, but almost six years later, it is a distant blur and just a blip on the radar, as my oncologist said to me at the beginning. You have such a positive attitude and an abundance of support and love from family and friends."

Camille chimed in: "Love the photo! I know that the prep on Monday will be no picnic. Tuesday will be here before you know it and you will be in that lovely hospital gown which is always too short. Well Chuck, this is my prayer for your doctor: May the Healing Christ bless him with compassion and excellence. For you, may Christ give to you His peace in your soul, His presence in your heart, His power in your recovery. Even though I am not Irish, here is another good wish: May God's blessings outnumber the shamrocks that grow!"

Jim Vedro added. "Hello Charles (always so formal) Great picture of a fine couple. The Sunday morning Eucharist sounded like a profound religious experience and the assurance you walk with God. He will lead you onto your surgery with inner peace. Stay strong in the Lord and all who care about you."

Aunt May also loved the picture. She was glad to be at the anointing in spirit. She is anxious to know the time of surgery (ME TOO!)

Frank Berge (another friend and classmate): "Prayerful love to you both. Have been remembering you with our fondest prayerful best wishes and will join the chorus of Holy Men and Women raising their voices in prayer on Tuesday."

On Monday, March 21st posting was at 3:41 AM–wonder why I couldn't sleep? Not much to add after yesterday's detailed posting. I was looking forward to going to work for the last time. I do know that Burger King was the least of my worries as I am leaving it in the capable hands of Eileen, the best general manager I have ever had. My Burger King family is so special to me. They really are my extended family. I ended the posting by saying, "You will all be with me over the next 48 hours. I will be smiling and singing, "Be not afraid, I go before you always. Come follow me and I will give you rest."

Yet again, I am overwhelmed by everyone's support. It is the only way I could get through it all. Nineteen entries on CB, countless emails, and many phone calls–wow! Thank You. Many of the CB entries were well-wishers for a speedy recovery including, Anne Stehle, Anne Michels, Mary Kuli, Gwen (who is praying for miracles), Theresa, and Frank Berge.

Camille made fun of my bowling. She adds: "Even though there is no sun this morning, I know you are listening to God speak to you; and it's like sitting in the sun because, "The Lord is my light and salvation, of whom should I be afraid?"

Aunt May wrote: "May today pass quickly as you enjoy your special diet. I'm asking the dear Lord to continue holding you in the palm of His hand as He has for the past 59 years. Let the sun shine inside and out." *Funny how my aunt and Camille both referred to the sun – they are bonded together in more ways than one.*

Wonderful Sr. Betty reminded us that she is "with you in prayer. You will be remembered in our evening Mass tonight. You are surrounded and held by grace."

Joan Walsh challenged me to "Stay strong and keep the faith. I along with so many others will be sending you positive thoughts and energy all day tomorrow. May the good saints protect you today, tomorrow, and ever after. And may troubles ignore you each step of the way.

Sr. Marge wrote: "Your news continues to be hopeful and

encouraging. You and your caring team of doctors and nurses are in my prayers. I rejoice that you can draw strength from each of us who care about you. You will be in my prayers tomorrow afternoon during the surgery. May all go well and may complete healing and renewed energy be a gift from God."

Cousin Joannie wrote that tomorrow my unwanted boarder will be evicted for good.

Competitive Ellen said, "Sooo glad tomorrow is almost here! I am very much looking forward to 5:00 when you are cancer free. Thankfully I will be there all day with you. When they take you back for surgery, just think of me beating Matt, Ryan, and mom in cards … I know that will make you smile! Can't wait until you come home so I can beat YOU in cards … and bowling!! Seriously though, I have every bit of confidence that you will beat this!! All of OUR many, many prayers will be answered."

My cancer buddy Janie is looking forward to seeing me so that we can do the Happy Dance together. She told me to "be brave and keep smiling."

Aunt May got on again to let me know that she has now placed Dr. Hafez on the prayer list with her community. She wants him to know that "80 Sisters of St. Joseph will be praying for him and the guidance of his hands. Dr. Hafez will be prayed for at the 11:00 AM Mass and the 4:00 PM community prayer." And then she kiddingly reminded me that I am still on that prayer list too.

Peggy said: "Good riddance to that pesky cancer."

My niece Denise expressed her confidence that everything will go great. "The worst will be behind you VERY SOON! *Aren't those nieces and nephews something else?!*

My friend Bev Beltramo wrote today. She is the head chaplain over all of the Oakwood Hospitals and is always supportive. Her wisdom for the day was, "we cannot choose the things that happen to us, but we can chose how we respond." She is not sure who wrote it, but it sure fits. "I know you sure as heck would not have chosen THIS, but you are sure making choices as to how you respond; reaching out to those who care about you, keeping a positive spirit, allowing God to walk beside you and give you strength."

And the best entry of the day from the Jaskulas:
"HAIL TO THE VICTORS!"

Chapter Eight
My All-Inclusive Trip to U of M
March 22-25

Tuesday, March 22, I wrote my first post of the day at 3:31 a.m.; Not sure why I was having a hard time sleeping. "If you listen real close you can probably hear the trumpets: "Celebrate good times! Come on! It is a day to celebrate. An old high school buddy (Bill Bouie) wrote that today is his birthday and said, "I am the most blessed man that has ever been born and your successful surgery will be a great gift." In many ways today is like a birthday for me--a birth into new life. And I have to disagree with Bill because I feel like I am the most blessed man ever born. When Ellen allowed me to speak at her wedding (sort of), I concluded my comments by saying, "Can you feel the love?" Well I have felt all of your love and prayers these last 35 days and would be lost without it. In many ways my cancer is ever so slight. All of us have stories about people in much more difficult situations, including death. I met a man yesterday with cancer in his eye. I am thrilled to move forward today, my new birthday. I have to close by singling out my ROCK, Jeannie. She has been incredible these last 35 days. She has kept me busy to avoid the lows I have experienced. How does she handle her lows?? When she pledged her unconditional love on August 24, 1979, she had no clue about today. Thanks, Rock. I love you ever so much. Celebrate the good times. God is good.

At 6:09 AM I had a second entry – short and sweet in large letters: GOD BLESS DR. HAFEZ

Right after the second posting I took a relaxing shower. U of M leaves nothing for the imagination. Their instructions are very thorough. Not only did they say to use a non-scented soap/shampoo, they specifically identified that the preferred soap was Dial. Not wanting to upset anything, I went to CVS yesterday and bought a two-pack of Dial. Do not ask why I bought a 2 pack for one shower, but I am still using it.

Camille went to Mass this morning and talked with Fr. Pat Halfpenny, her pastor. He is a contemporary of mine from seminary days and also presented me the seminary's Alumni of the Year award in 1989. He prayed for me, the doctor, the nurses, and promised to be with me in prayer throughout the day. She added that he did say a beautiful prayer for me.

I also called Aunt May at about 6:00 AM so she could be reassured by my voice – not sure who was reassuring whom. Aunt May sent a CB message at 7:19 and Camille sent one at 7:17 – it is amazing how often their messages come at close times and have similar content.

7:30 AM:

We arrived at Gabriel Richard for Mass. Jeannie, Ellen, Matt, Ryan and I sat together in the back. Fr. Bob McCabe celebrates Mass for GR students every Tuesday and does a fine job. After Mass, he came up and hugged me and wished me well. At the conclusion of Mass, Joe Whalen asked all of the students to sit down. He told the story about how important it is for families to share with each other. He then talked about my cancer and asked the student body to rise. They joined hands and we prayed the Lord's Prayer together – a little sobbing for sure. At the conclusion he said, "We love you Chuck and good luck." Pretty interesting from a man I didn't know six months ago.

8:30-9:30 AM:

What a ride to U of M. Many times there was complete silence, as we dwelled on our personal innermost thoughts. And then we would say something silly to cut through the quiet. Ellen's mother-in-law called to assure me of her prayers – yet another person on our team.

9:30 AM:

Our caravan descended on U of M. We went to the check-in area, very quiet and serene. The lady behind the desk asked me if I knew what I was checking in for (I guess that is routine). I jokingly said that

I was checking in for my three-day all-inclusive vacation. Everybody within ear shot smiled. I then had to fill out medical records AGAIN, for the last time. They gave us a beeper, kind of like what you get at Outback Steakhouse (I hadn't eaten in two days) and told us it would be about 11:00 when I was called back. The problem with the pager is that we were not at a restaurant and I WAS THE MAIN COURSE. I was anxious and couldn't sit still. I began to pace the halls. I bet I walked over five miles that day. Jeannie said the janitors were mad because the place will need a new wax job. I also wore out a new pair of shoes, but it was better than sitting and playing cards with Ellen. Jeannie located a computer in the lounge to do up-to-the-minute CB updates. There was a porter in the lounge area offering folks drinks. I gladly accepted until Ellen reminded everyone that I had to abstain.

10:59 PM:

I gathered the family together and went to the hallway to pray the Lord's Prayer together. They wrapped their arms around me and we left room in the middle for everyone else. "Can you feel the love?" And the beeper did NOT go off. I usually am prompt, so I was disappointed that the beeper was quiet. So nothing else to do, but walk and wait for the beep. *Might be a great time to say the Lord's Prayer right now for some special intention in your life!*

12:00 PM:

I went to check-in desk to get an update. They explained that there were problems with the morning surgery and that Dr. Hafez was still operating. He had warned me on Sunday that the early surgery was a complicated surgery, so I was not surprised. Time for a brief prayer for that patient. More walking.

12:30 PM:

I had promised Joey that he would be my phone call right before I went back; now seemed to be a good time for that call. Throughout this journey I did speak daily with Joe. I really wished he could be here, but it made more economic sense for him to stay in Vegas. So we chatted for a bit before I went back.

12:45 p.m.:

I ran out of things to say with Joe so we disconnected; hard to believe I was speechless. But still no buzzer, so I decided to call Eileen and check in with Burger King. I do not have a clue what we talked about, but then the buzzer started beeping. I was crying and said good-bye.

1:00 PM:

I went back to begin my final preparation, a long-awaited moment. I kissed my kids and hugged them furiously. Jeannie was allowed back with me. Thank God. The nurse admonished me for not removing my wedding ring; I have worn it for so long it seems like part of my hand. They had a tough time getting it off, but finally had success. More questions – did I say more questions? Dr. Hafez came by to say hello. I was glad to see him. We visited and he looked over my abdomen. Then he pulled out an orange Sharpee from his lab coat, drew a line on my right side, and initialed it. It is his responsibility to mark the spot of the incision and then he is legally obligated to initial it. Even for this surgery there are rules.

There were two options for pain control. One was an epidural in the back, but they were skeptical if that would work because it did not work with the Whipple surgery. The other option was a morphine drip. The problem with the morphine drip was that at the time of the Whipple, it was the avenue we took, and the morphine really made me loopy – I hated it. So we discussed it for a while and thought we would try the epidural again. This time it worked!!

Family strikes again. The surgical nurse in charge of my case, could have been my nephew's, Mikey's, twin. As we were all a tad nervous, it was a great ice breaker, we even called the guy Mike. Always time for a little humor, even at a time like this.

Jeannie kept using the computer in the lounge to update everyone on CB; what a great convenience they provided.

3:30 PM:

Let's get this show on the road. Jeannie came back to say good bye. We asked Dr. Hafez how long the surgery would take. He responded that he had booked the room for four-and-a-half hours. He did say, "The surgery will take as much time as needed." He wasn't saying that sarcastically, but he hates to predict anything and then frustrate his patients and their families. I kissed my bride and was rolled away. I glanced down the hall and saw the kids, gave then a wave, and a thumbs up ("thumbs up" is kind of a trademark – it was the sign I gave Jeannie when I got out of the Whipple surgery and I plan on using it later today!).

4:00 PM:

Dr. Hafez washed his hands, after he shook mine and gave me reassuring comments. I can still see him standing at the sink and that is the last this I remember of the day.

For the next two-and-a-half hours, Ellen dominated everyone with her card skills. They had a bite to eat, but other than Matt, nobody was very hungry. One of Ellen's good buddies, Stephanie Pease, lives near the hospital. She stopped by to visit. It was a tension reliever and much appreciated. Matt, my incessant text messager, was receiving messages form his buddies. It seems every teacher at GR started every class with a prayer for Mr. Pio – what a helluva family.

6:30 PM:

SURGERY WAS SUCCESSFUL!!! Was there any doubt? I was pleased that it only took two and-a-half hours, since they had set aside four and-a-half hours – absolutely no complications. Glad I was easy. The tumor was on top of the kidney and very easy to remove. They did not have to give me any blood, not that I would have known.

I was in the recovery room for the next two hours, but have absolutely no memory of it at all. Jeannie could not rave enough about the care of those nurses. One would expect nothing but the best from U of M and Jeannie assures me that was the case. Hail to the Victors!!

8:30 PM:

Finally got admitted to my room. I was still out of it, but I do remember being able to give each of my awesome family a hug one by one and then they headed for home. I had a very restful night. Don't remember much, but I do know one thing. At 3:00 AM, they came to draw my blood, as they would at the same time every night/morning. Couldn't they leave this job for the day shift? I am really "sawing logs" and have to wake up to be pricked by a vampire. Oh well, can't stand in the way of modern medicine.

I will not even try to enumerate all of the calls, emails, and CB messages. If Jeannie answered them all, she would just about be finishing up. The only one that Jeannie could not respond to was from Andy Garlic, he wrote the darn thing in Latin; "Custodiant et Sancti et Angelia ab omnibus malis!" Where is Fr. Walker when you need him? *Thanks all of you who prayed that day and every day!*

Wednesday, March 23rd:

Today would have been my dad's 92nd birthday. Happy Birthday, Hank. Had he been alive we would have probably been eating pineapple upside down cake. Yum! And I am still on a liquid diet.

Jeannie started the day with an incredible CB entry. She stated: "Good morning, what a beautiful sight to see my best friend's beautiful blue eyes! Charlie looks great but tired. Already went for two walks by the time I got to U of M. He is resting now, but thinks he should go home tomorrow. Thanks again for the warm thoughts and wonderful prayers." *Jeannie truly is MY best friend. I was truly moved by this email; very simple yet poetic.*

Joe Whalen (friend and boss) sent an email to us today in response to the above CB entry. Turns out he, too, was quite moved by Jeannie's poetic statements. When he read the comments he said it moved him to tears as well. I guess we are all a bunch of crybabies. *I can't tell you how many times I have been crying while I have been writing this.* I so appreciate Joe's support. He is not just my wife's boss, he is our friend. And what a principal he will be for the resurgence of Gabriel Richard.

Today is my first full day in the hospital. Much of what I will write about the next three days is information that others have told me, as the pain medications that were administered to me left me in a fog. Jeannie went to work, but the school had planned to give her the day off and had prearranged a sub so she could spend it with me; how thoughtful. When she got to the hospital, I was just returning from my first walk. The intern working with Dr. Hafez told me I have to walk six times and sit in the chair three times. Neither of these items was on my: "want to do list", but I knew they were mandatory before I could plan my great escape. I always follow doctor's orders. By the time Jeannie left at 6:30 PM I had accomplished those goals. Mid-morning the chaplain came to bring communion, which was very welcomed. Of course, I evaluated the quality of his presence since it is how I spend every Thursday. It was great that he was there, but it seemed like he was on a mission to get his list complete; it was a good lesson for me to make sure that each visit I make is a quality visit.

Ron Victor came for a visit; long way for him to come from Roseville. It sure was good to see him. He also brought communion. What the heck, if one dose of the Eucharist in the day is fulfilling, just imagine what two does. *Funny thing is that I sadly did not remember Ron's visit. I guess I was sociable, but it wasn't until I began to work on this book that I had a recall of his being there.* It is great to have a priest in the "family."

I had four other visitors that day. Ellen and Matt came up after school. Ellen was disappointed that I was not up for a game of cards. Guess she'll have to beat herself in solitaire. Also coming in were Brother Steve and cousin Joanie. A little explanation about Brother Steve – Steve is my sister-in-law's (Barb Pio's) brother. Rather trying to explain all of that, we lovingly refer to him as Brother Steve. Any time you see him he is wearing two things: a huge smile and a Hawaiian shirt. They came to support me as well. *Sadly, like Ron Victor, I did not remember JoAnne being there until I began working on this book. It does amaze me how powerful drugs are. Just the other day I met a woman who was bragging about being "clean" due to an addiction to prescription drugs – so sad, but so real.*

Medically, my sugar is way out of whack, but that is normal following surgery. They check my levels frequently and are always ready with a shot of insulin. Dr. Hafez stopped by for a brief visit, looked at the incision and is thrilled with how well the surgery went. He is a busy man, sad to say it would be the last time I would see him until the end of July. I was History, and he had many other miracles to perform. He indicated that I will either go home late Thursday or on Friday.

My diet is a total liquid diet, which is understood; nonetheless, it is not very enjoyable. How much can one drink? But they are slowly waking up my insides, as I have had nothing to eat since Elaine Simon's lemon meringue pie on Sunday.

In her CB entry that day, Jeannie complained about how cold the hospital was. Jeannie is never cold and I am always cold – good to have the shoe on the other foot for a change.

As you can imagine, many more CB entries for Jeannie to go through this evening. Most of them I will not list as there is not enough paper. Suffice it to say everyone is breathing easier *(ME TOO!)* I found it interesting that three new people entered something today. Turns out they have been following all along, but never entered until today. Jeremy Bergman manages a Burger King that Jeannie, Matt, and I frequent every Thursday morning for breakfast. It is a nice routine and always good to visit with Jeremy. Gregg Shields is another seminary buddy who I frequently visit with on a baseball blog, At the Corner. In fact, if you like talking baseball, consider joining us. Gregg simply summed it all up by saying, "Better days are coming." Jeannie's brother, Chuck, also chimed in and continues to pray. So nice to have so much support.

Thursday, March 24th:

A beautiful day in the neighborhood! *God has blessed me with the gift of another day – one of my new habits is that as I wake each day I say: "Thanks, God, for the gift of another day!" Try it!*

The commissary staff brought my wonderful liquid breakfast. It is easy to complain about it, but I still don't have much of an appetite. The nurses are still telling me I have to walk, every time I can. The more I walk, the quicker I can go home; so off I went.

When I came back to the hotel room, I dropped something and bent over to pick it up without thinking. It was a natural instinctive motion. As I put my head down to look and pick up the item, I got lightheaded instantly and knew I was in trouble. In no time I fell over. Ouch! Now what! I knew that I was in a lot of pain, but felt there was nothing seriously wrong. The spot where the IV was inserted was throbbing. Because I had just gotten back from a walk, I had no access to the nurse's call button. Even if I had, I don't know if I would have used it; pride is a strange thing. Even if I had no physical injuries, my pride was definitely hurt and I didn't need anyone to know. So I laid there in a heap, thinking. I had no strength as I had just walked. I couldn't get up. Finally I could drag over a chair with my foot and then I could pull myself up using that chair. Relief and success. How scary. I know I will follow a different routine in the future if I drop something.

Just as I got into bed, a nurse walked in. Perfect timing! I decided to be honest and tell her what had happened. She checked me over and pronounced me fit as a fiddle. What happened next was pretty amazing. The nurse (Mary) was wearing a multi-colored button that said "Live." My curiosity got the best of me and I asked Mary what the button meant. She pulled up a chair and sat down. She explained that she has two grown daughters. One of them is leading a "traditional and normal life." The other daughter is gay. Mary then spent the next hour talking about the amount of abuse her daughter has taken due to her choice to have announced her choice of sexuality. Mary wears that button because she feels her daughter deserves the same opportunities that we all receive. She graphically described several occasions of abuse. It was a very moving message. In her own simple way, by wearing that button, Mary is trying to do her best to help move the world forward. Hurray for Mary! That conversation certainly impacted me, and I can see her now. Abuse of any form is nasty and should not be tolerated, whatever the situation is. Have I been guilty of abuse? Have you? Are we open-minded? Verbal abuse? Making fun of others? Race and sexual orientation seem to be easy targets, but why? This incident, and the thinking that went with it, will make me a better person.

Shortly after Mary left, the Hospital's Eucharistic Minister approached. Today's bearer of Christ was much more engaging than yesterday's. He sat down and we had quite a conversation. It is amazing how much you can share with somebody when you have the common bond of Jesus. It was interesting because I had just fallen and then had spent an hour with Mary. I shared those two incidents with the minister. He, too, appreciated the impact both of those incidents had.

Once the minister left, I dozed off and on and waited for Jeannie and Matt. We all love all of our kids, but Matt has been so special throughout this ordeal. From the moment he learned of the cancer through today, he has truly walked with me. He is a hugger and I was the recipient of many warm hugs and expressions of love. Thanks Matt!!

At lunch time they brought me more fluids. I explained to the lady from the commissary, that the nurse had recently put me on a regular diet. She looked at me quite disbelievingly. Her body language said, "Yea, right!" I said that I was serious. I asked her to please double check. She was gone for an hour (seemed like it). She finally returned with the coveted FOOD. I removed the lid, looked at the food, and asked her to leave the liquid diet, as I was more apt to drink that than eat what she had brought. Hospital food is legendary.

Right after lunch I began to receive some welcomed visitors. The first two were Susie and Rich, two of my employees. They even brought along a beautiful plant. It was special that they took out time from their day to visit. I have often talked about the relationship I hope to establish with my employees as one of a family and Rich and Susie proved it!

Then Aunt May, Sr. Jeanne Lenora, and Sr. Marge drove in from Kalamazoo. As I have written earlier, what a bond I have with those sisters. I was moved that they were willing to make that long trip to spend time with me. Sr. Jeanne has been Aunt May's friend for years. My kids also love her. She has some physical challenges, but she did not let her infirmities stop her from this special visit. As neither my aunt nor Sr. Jeanne drive any more, Sr. Marge was elected taxi driver. Pretty impressive that the head of the community took time out of her packed schedule to be with me--impressive and humbling! We had a delightful and lively conversation. Don't ask me about what happened during the visit because the drugs were still dominating my body, but I loved their visit. Jeannie and Matt arrived and we all laughed a lot. Thank God for private rooms.

The nuns left for their return trip to Kalamazoo, and Jeannie, Matt, and I reviewed the day. Jeannie, who I have begun to lovingly call "The Warden," realized that I had been entertaining all afternoon and so I had not walked. "Up and at 'em," she commanded. This walk was easier as they had removed the IV earlier and I no longer needed to walk with that pole. While we were walking, we were joined by my restaurant manager and friend, Eileen. It was great to see her, but embarrassing, as she too has a very busy schedule, especially in light of my absence. I continue to be humbled by visits, CB entries, emails, cards, and people just expressing their love.

Jeannie and Matt left early (is there a schedule?) as it was Matt's basketball banquet. As I was frustrated with this basketball season, I was glad to have a good excuse to be absent. Once again, the Lord reminded me to not be so judgmental. The coach chose to begin the banquet in prayer for my speedy recovery. That was not necessary, but certainly appreciated. Jeannie would later write that: "It was a great testimony for my wonderful husband." She is so amazingly strong and kind – she can still call me wonderful despite everything I have dragged her through.

Once all of my company left, the real highlight of the day came, the removal of the catheter. Catheters are necessary evils. But really! The nurse painfully removed it and I was instantly relieved. She warned me of the need for me to go as soon as possible so that the staff would realize that my plumbing is OK. At 7:00 PM, a crusty night nurse (she was only doing her job) informed me that I had one more hour to go or they would reinsert the catheter. That was not gonna happen. I looked at the remainder of the fluids on my dinner tray and began to wonder how close they would inspect the sample I would leave. A plan was hatched. 8:00 PM came and went and no inspector came in, nor was I able to produce. I finally had a little success at 9:00, but no nurse ever came in to check. I guess their scare tactics were successful.

Once again there were so many expressions of love that day on CB. When Matt got to school that day, one of his buddies said, "How's the King?" It is so impressive to be walking with the GR community. The well wishes continued. One of my customers (Jim Vibbart) even chimed in his support. I shouldn't even call him a customer. So many of my customers have become life-long friends.

Chris Lees, a fellow volunteer at Southshore Hospital, cautioned me to not rush it. She reminded me that I was still needed at Southshore

– nice to be needed and reminded of it.

Friday, March 25th:

The day I have been waiting for, Get away day. Camille wrote on CB what a wonderful word "HOME" is! Amen! Like they said in that wonderful movie, <u>The Wizard of Oz,</u> there's no place like home! Mary (the nurse I have bonded with from yesterday) came in and gave me the word that I could go home. She sat down in the chair and went through my discharge instructions and had me sign them. We also talked a little more about her daughter's struggles and I assured her that her daughter will always have a place in my prayers. *Sad to say, "Out of sight, out of mind" comes in to play here. Once I left the hospital my time was filled with a healthy recovery, and I actually forgot about Mary and her daughter. Writing this book has rekindled that memory. I prayed for Mary and her daughter today, and will be reminded every time I reread this book.* It was now 10:00 AM and I was packing. I called Jeannie to share the good news with her. She knew she couldn't come until after school. I told her that was fine. I knew I was getting out and all I had was time. I finished packing and spent some of the time reading. Much of the rest of the time was spent in prayer--prayers of thanksgiving for the fine work of Dr. Hafez and his team of experts, prayers for my wonderful extended family, prayers for The Warden, and prayers for Mary and her daughter. I was anxious to leave, so I figured I would save Jeannie some time. I called the transportation department and asked them to deliver a wheel chair to the room. I was proudly sitting in that chariot when Jeannie arrived. I said, "Let's go home!" That sounded great. Jeannie started to push the nurse's call button. I told her that was not necessary. I said they brought the wheel chair because they were giving Jeannie permission to push me to the car. Jeannie was perplexed and said that any hospital she had ever heard of always demanded that they push you out for insurance liability purposes. I told her that was not the case at U of M. I told her that I had signed myself out earlier. I must have been convincing because we were on our way. Once Jeannie figured out I may have told a little white lie, she was not happy. She commented that was the last time she would ever believe a drugged-up patient.

Chapter Nine

The Beginning of Recovery
The rest of March

Friday, March 25th, *4:00 PM:*

I got home and collapsed into bed. I had no idea how draining the car ride home could be. Collapsing into bed was easier said than done. I had been instructed by the nurses that I could not lay on my right side, where the incision was, for now. As it had been designated 31 ½ years ago, I am to sleep on the left side of the bed, with no exceptions. Somehow I got in the right position and promptly slept – a lot. The only time I woke up was when the Warden came in to see if I was ok or to administer some medication. My recollection was that night went pretty smooth. I just know I was thrilled to be home and begin the next phase of my recovery.

Saturday, March 26th:

After a fitful night's rest, I was ready to tackle my first full day at home. I still had no appetite, but the Warden insisted I eat. I did manage to enjoy two poached eggs and two sausages. Then I slept for a couple of hours. Thankfully, there is a recliner next to my bed, so I was able to sit up and eat. After breakfast, Jeannie printed off all of the amazing comments from CB so that I could read them, and I cried and cried. Joy commented on how wonderful it was to have a supportive community, which it is. Thanks to all for their support and comments.

Bill Bouie kind of rubbed it in when he said: "Keep charging my friend and you will be back as good as new in no time. Wish that I was there to visit, but I am in Florida watching our Tigers for you. They look pretty good and very determined." That was good news to me. As I plan to watch a lot of the Tigers during this summer, I was glad to know that they looked good. Looking good and determined sounds like a great goal for me, too.

One of my first challenges comes in the form of pain medicine. The only way I can drive and move this recovery process quicker is to be off the pain medicine. However, I have so much pain, it is unbearable. The IV did a great job in the hospital, but I am home now, and don't have that option. I know that there is no need to drive for a while, but I always plan ahead. OCD? I gladly take the narcotic for relief, but I do wonder to myself, when can I move on to just aspirin?

The Warden was on patrol and made me walk. She wanted me to go outside, but I told her that I couldn't – maybe the proper word was wouldn't. Anyhow, she commanded that I walk inside the house, two times around the stairs, through the kitchen and dining room; two was fine. She wanted three, but I won out. I did eat some strawberries and mandarin oranges to satisfy her wishes.

An awesome and humiliating moment came tonight. I finally got a real shower. I have had plenty of sponge baths, but no real showers. As I anticipated this shower, I realized how much of an invalid I am. Jeannie had to do much of the work, but man oh man, what a feeling to be squeaky clean!! The shower will be a highlight of my evenings.

Sunday, March 27th:

I began the day having oatmeal with strawberries in it. I have not eaten much, and what I have eaten has not stayed with me. Not to sound graphic, but vomiting is not a pleasure for anyone. Imagine me, in my unstable state, positioning myself in front of the toilet, to deposit my meals. The pain I experienced each time I wretched was unbelievable. My right side just throbbed. This is recovery, welcome to my world!

The Warden informed me that I am going outside today to walk. It is a sunny day and there is no excuse to stay inside. Kris Jaskula commented that my smiling face added to the sunny day. Believe me, I was not smiling at the thought of walking, but was smiling as this was progress! My mind went to work, but I came up with no good reasons not to walk outside. I have to admit it was great to go outside, and it was a great personal triumph. We only walked the length of two houses, but it was the next step.

We had our first company today. It was special for the Simons and Jaskulas to come over. As you might recall, Elaine Simon was the first person to offer a rosary for my intention, followed by many of you – especially Fr. Prus on his daily walk. As I do not own a rosary it is impossible for me to reciprocate. Not a problem anymore. The Simons gifted me with an awesome rosary, my first since my First Communion. What a priceless treasure. And in the past few months I fervently work those beads. When I can't sleep at night, I crawl into that recliner and use the rosary. Jeannie chuckles as she can hear those beads at work, I hope I haven't awakened her too often.

Bev Beltramo commented on CB: "My goodness – I know why you're so tired – 15 pages of notes in this guestbook! That's a day's work just to read it all. Guess people must kinda care about you, eh? All that care and concern and love is pretty darn good medicine, so hope to see you tap dancing down the hallway soon! Isn't it a miracle the ways God takes these really awful things and turns them into opportunities for us to receive blessings? Only God could do that! (Of course our job is to notice and sometimes that is not a small thing!)" *Thank you Bev, what a great summary of this experience. Your words are a reminder and a true prayer.*

Things are moving forward. Jeannie and the rest of my team went bowling tonight. Matt is left in charge. I was feeling a little brave and so I asked Matt to take me for a second walk today while Jeannie was bowling and he gladly obliged. I know that the more I exercise, the faster my recovery will progress, so I have to challenge myself daily! Jeannie came home thrilled that she had rolled four strikes in a row, even brought in the score sheet to prove it. I am looking for more improvement tomorrow, with my recovery and not just Jeannie's bowling.

Monday, March 28th:

Jeannie's CB entry: "I am hoping to get Charlie on a THREE house walk today. He still has no appetite but I guess since he is not doing anything this would be normal. I am trying to get him to eat before he takes his medicine to cut down on the nausea. I pray for each of you daily, thanks so much for you prayers." Leave it to Jeannie to make sure that she prays for all of you in her spare time. Prayer is a much more important part of our lives.

Jeannie spoils me each morning with breakfast in the reclining chair. It is oatmeal with whatever fruit she has in the house and a glass of Hawaiian Punch. I used to love that punch as a kid, but no longer drink it, mostly due to the high sugar content. I probably should not be drinking it now either, but it tastes good and it stays with me. And I am eating. Mid-afternoon we did get in that THREE house walk.

Tuesday, March 29th: A sad day for me. Jeannie went back to work. I didn't admit it then (and she probably won't know until she reads this entry), but I was nervous. Could I make it alone? I have become pretty dependent, so it is a good thing she went back to work. I did fine by myself. She made breakfast and got me situated in the living room. She put a peanut butter and jelly sandwich in a lunch bag so I had lunch prepared. I am having a hard time drinking anything, even just water. I know that is necessary for recovery, but it ain't happening. When Jeannie got home from school I put my coat on and walked four houses. Recovery is happening, just not fast enough for me.

We continue to draw on the strength of all our loved ones from CB. Today there was a new author, Jane Paris, Jeannie's friend from years ago. We heard from another state, North Carolina. Joanne Schigelone jokingly referred to Jeannie as the "drill sergeant," as confirmed by her two sons who Jeannie has taught.

Wednesday, March 30th:

Different day, same routine. I am proud to say that I add another house each day as I walk, building up stamina. Three interesting CB entries today.

Cathy Bernhold told me to watch the Price is Right and also told me to avoid soap operas. I do not have the attention span to read and I have learned quickly that TV is useless. I can't wait for the Tigers season to begin. I am still sleeping a lot so the time passes when Jeannie is at school. She comes home, we walk, and then I sleep.

Sr. Betty wrote that: "We are all given opportunities to learn the lessons we need, like patience! (*She knows me too well – patience – yuk.*) Please take this a day at a time and a step at a time as you move into greater health. It is all soul work, you know."

We also heard from Jackie Sheridan. She is a fellow volunteer at Southshore. She offered her support and promised continued prayers for both of us. *What makes this interesting is that I am writing this page the day after Jackie's husband's funeral. What an awesome spirit Charlie had. He spent the last 51 years of his life in a wheel chair, following a motor cycle accident. Charlie never let his physical disability get in the way. Anything was possible for Charlie. He truly was an inspiration. At his funeral, the priest talked about how easy it is for handicapped people to be overlooked, but those of us without physical limitations have the real handicap between our ears.* So here is Jackie supporting us and three and-a-half months later we are praying with her for Charlie; it is a small world.

Chapter Ten

Recovery Continues
April 1–14

Friday, April 1st:

Happy April Fool's Day! No joking for me, just a continuation of celebrating LIFE! In celebration of this day, I was able to return to the keyboard. I wrote on CB: "Recovery is going as smooth as it should, just not fast enough to please this stubborn Polack. I have been cancer-free for ten days now – what a relief. Can't wait until I can say I have been pain-free for ten days. There still is lots of pain in right side. And where there is no pain, there is complete numbness. We go on Monday to have the staples removed which is another step in the right direction. I still do not have much of an appetite, but that will come back, I am sure. My personal goal is to get off the narcotic pain pill. I now take them every six hours, instead of four – I have to admit that sixth hour is really tough. And I plan to go on Tylenol really soon and totally get away from the narcotic. I am smiling and shaking my head right now – over 2,000 visits from my extended family to this CB website – that is incredible. I will never be able to repay all of your kindnesses and support – BUT I WILL TRY TO!"

I also remembered that today was the burial of Aunt Lorraine. She quietly passed away after suffering with Alzheimer's disease, complicated at the end with some physical problems. Her three kids (Lynn Marie, Mary Jo, and Tom) and their families have done a phenomenal job providing for her care. God Bless Lorraine Costello. I was unable to attend her funeral, it was a huge disappointment for me, but my body just is not ready.

My brother TR and Barb did come in town for the funeral. And that was good for me as I have not seen him since the surgery and that gave us a chance to visit. I have continued to talk to him daily, but it is not as good as seeing him and exchanging a bear hug – he just can't squeeze too hard yet. Of course, he tried too! We had an awesome visit. He demanded to go for a walk, my longest walk yet. I know I have to do this daily and to challenge myself to increase the amounts. I think I surprised TR with the distance I could endure, because at one point he wanted to turn around. He didn't think I could make the return trip. His visits are never long enough and he went home right after the funeral.

As you can imagine, lots of kind comments about my return to the keyboard. Bill Bouie was concerned that yesterday's Tiger loss might slow down my recovery. It didn't, but was a disappointment. At least there is finally something worthwhile to watch on TV. Pat Gonyea reminded me that her husband and I both turn 60 in October and we plan to party, so I have to be ready. Pat, being much older, has already reached that milestone.

Saturday, April 2nd:

More rest – it seems that is all I do.

Brother Steve came down for a visit. It was great to be with him. I asked him to give Jeannie a break and take me for a walk, as I am not steady enough to go by myself. He was happy to oblige. Half way through the walk we hit a snow/hail storm. There was no way I could run, so we continued on our merry way and just laughed. Jeannie was ready to come and find us, but we made it. My walks are no longer measured, they are just progress. Steve brought along some home-made sausage from some small store in Southwest Detroit. It was yummy and helped increase my appetite.

The daily CB intake included a comment from Aunt May admonishing me not to rush the healing process. The Berges talked about the generosity of love. Joy responded to my comment about wanting to repay everyone. She said there is never a need for me to repay her. I know that, but I know I will always be there for anyone who needs me.

Sunday, April 3rd:

I am still not well enough to go to church. I do miss it! I do get up by 6:00 AM and turn on Channel 2's Mass for Shut-Ins. It is the best I can do. It was a quiet day. Two CB comments. One from my friend Jim Vibbart from Whitmore Lake. He said that if I keep doing what I am supposed to I will be bouncing off the walls in no time. Mentally I already am! Tom and Jill Renaud, long time Ozanam friends, chimed in with their support. At night, Jeannie went bowling and Matt and I walked. A good day!

Monday, April 4:

This was a looong day. We went to U of M to have the staples removed, 22 in all. I am a typical male and a wuss when it comes to pain. I was very nervous, but things went very smooth. Jeannie said the only times I winced was at the removal of the first and last staples. The nurse did a phenomenal job of keeping me talking (which isn't too hard), so I didn't feel anything. He then glued some steri-strips over the wound. He did such a good job that my T-shirt was glued to the strips. He raved about what an awesome healing job is taking place, for this I am grateful. He rated it an A+. Do you know how good that makes me feel? We probably overdid it a little on the way home, made a couple of stops, including my first meal out in quite a while. Got home, was in extreme pain and exhausted. Took some pain pills and slept the rest of the afternoon.

An interesting thing happened in the conversation with the nurse. He asked if I was ready for the changes in my life. I said I have already experienced a lot. He said he was not talking about physical changes, but mental ones. He went out to say that I have been the STAR in everyone's life since the cancer discovery. Now as I am slipping back into normal life, the glow of the star will diminish. I will become an everyday guy and not at the top of everyone's prayer list. It is reality. It is another lesson of humility. It was something I had not thought of, but it is true. It is the way it should be. It is part of the life cycle; other folks now have greater needs with which we all have to concern ourselves. I really appreciated this revelation.

On Friday the 15th, I have an appointment with the Wizard, Dr.

Hafez. He will personally check out my progress. I am concerned about the numbness on the right side and will quiz him. I have lost another ten pounds, but I am not eating. The staff has encouraged me that when I do eat, I should eat lots of protein – chicken, fish, and eggs.

My emotional state is still interesting. I cry all of the time. I am still in awe of Jeannie and her constant loving support.

I closed the day by remembering our dear friend, Sr. Jeanne Lenora. A short time ago she made the trip from Kalamazoo to see me and now she is in Borgess Hospital suffering. Pray for her.

Joan Walsh commented on CB. She, too, is a cancer survivor. She said that having staples is better than stitches, as they tend to heal faster. Yeah! She told me not to worry about the numbness; nerves have been tampered with and they act funny as a result. She talked about my positive attitude. Many times I don't feel so positive, but when I hear things like that, I challenge myself to stay positive. She commented on Borgess Hospital. Seems that her husband, Rick, was once a patient there and his care was awesome. Small world. I commented about Sr. Jeanne, and Joan comes along and affirms the goodness of Borgess. We are all in this together.

My sister-in-law, Peggy, commented that perhaps I should consider drinking Herbal Life shakes. How can somebody whose nickname is Bones know anything about those shakes?

Tuesday, April 5th, was a routine day. I didn't even take the time to write in my CB journal. Aunt May did, though, surprise. She has written in that guestbook practically daily, and has those other sisters praying fervently as she prints off my journal entries and posts them for all to see. She commented that Jeannie is my nurse and my hero. Amen to that. She challenged me because I had written that I was not in a hurry, but she knows that is not always true.

My neighbor, friend, and fellow cancer survivor (Jeannette) said she had stopped by to visit, but it never looks like I am up. I do spend a lot of time in the back bedroom, but I am always up for company. She said not to be bothered about the numbness, as it is much better to have that than what they removed. I am lucky that God has blessed me so.

Mary Kuli pointed out the great progress that I am having. I could not have dealt with having staples removed and making a few stops, just a week ago, so there is progress. She, too, included prayers for Sr. Jeanne.

Theresa said: "Slow and steady wins the race. I am proud of your progress! Both your and Jeannie's deep faith will keep you moving toward recovery." Theresa is such a dear. She teaches kindergarten at St. Mary's in Wayne. In addition to her personal powerful prayer, she had enlisted the aid of all of her students. Here are a bunch of kids, who I will never meet, that are taking time to remember me to Jesus. WOW!

Jane Paris, a close friend of Jeannie's commented on all of the work that Jeannie has done. She said, "Yes, poor Jeannie…now wait, knowing Jeannie I should say, "poor you!" I love you guys and wish I were nearer to shoot the breeze, or do schnapps shots – either works! My prayers and all the positive forces I can muster are with you!"

BUSTED #1: As I am getting stronger every day, I decided today was the day to shower alone. Had I asked permission from the Warden, I would surely have been denied. So I waited until she was busy on the computer and I cleaned up. As I was getting out of the shower to dry off, Jeannie realized that my room was quiet and she knew what I had done. I can still see her with her hands on her hips. She was concerned that I could have hurt myself. I didn't, and will no longer use her help in the shower. I have sure appreciated it, but time to move forward, another positive step.

Wednesday, April 6th:

Today I wrote that "patience is a virtue." Monday was extremely busy and Tuesday I could not get out of bed. Two steps forward and one step back. I am healed, but am waiting for the recovery to catch up. The highlight of the day was a visit from Mike and Cathy Morris. Mike and I are life-long friends. We stood up in each other's weddings. In fact, I introduced Mike to Cathy. They stopped in for a visit. I never got off the couch, but was so pleased to see them. They brought an awesome deli sandwich. They put it in the fridge for later. A couple hours later, I rolled off the couch to check it out. They put it right next to my daily peanut butter and jelly (Jeannie is way too good to me). I weighed the options and decided to tackle that deli treat. I could only eat half of it, but it was yummy.

It must have been seminary day today. Frank Berge called to offer his support. I also received a greeting card from Bill Sirois, a friend since Mt. Carmel days in fifth grade. How do people survive cancer without family, friends, and LOVE?

Thursday, April 7th:

I was up at 5:07 AM and I wrote the following on CB: "Had a great day yesterday. Watched our Tigers until 9:00 PM and couldn't keep my eyes open; figured they could win without me! Woke up wide awake at 1:30 a.m. Prayed the rosary for all of you for an hour and was still wide awake, so then I decided to finish that wonderful sandwich that the Morisses brought me and to finish the book I am reading. It is a biography about Lance Armstrong. It's not about the bike, <u>My Journey Back to Life.</u> It is a very penetrating book and one that I recommend everyone to read. A caution thought: Mr. Armstrong's language can be offensive. That is just his way of life. That being said, what a great story of victory. His cancer and treatment make mine look like a walk in the park. I called cancer a Beast; he chooses a different "B" word, but the effect is the same. I am in an astute club. I am a cancer survivor and darn proud of it. I have a bright future, and Bruce Gonyea and I plan to have an awesome 60th birthday in October. *And did we ever!! We rented a hall, had awesome guests, and a surprise visit from two of the finest clowns in the Downriver area; Bruce and I had rented clown costumes for the occasion. A good time was had by all.* Lance Armstrong writes: "If you get a second chance in life for something, you've got to go all the way." What an awesome thought. He later says: "If there is a purpose to the suffering that is cancer, I think it must be this: it's meant to improve us!" Shouldn't that be a great daily goal for all of us? TO IMPROVE!"

Some of the usual cast of characters weighed in on CB. Rick and Sheri are having a great life in California, celebrating 35 years of marriage this year. Tom Renaud introduced a mutual friend of ours and another Ozanam alumnus, Dave Howell to this website. Camille went to Mass this morning and Pat Halfpenny inquired as to my well-being, the length of relationships is amazing. Barb Koster was also inspired by Armstrong's book. She is an athlete, so it has an even stronger meaning for her. And Jeannie's friend, Fritzi, feels she has finally figured out the technology of CB. If I can get on that website it can't be too tough. Jane Paris wants to be at the 60th birthday party!!

Sunday, April 10th:

Day 13 of Recovery. By the fact that I have taken the time to count the days of recovery should give you an indication of how slowly I feel it is moving. Don't get me wrong, it is great to be cancer free, but I will not feel totally free of cancer until recovery moves along. I have good days followed by bad days which makes great sense, because on a good day I do too much so then the body revolts and the next day I am not able to do the simplest of tasks. The highlight of the week is that my son-in-law (still feels funny to have one of those) was nice enough to drive me to Burger King on Friday. Gosh did that feel great!! And the best part of it was that the staff did not know I was coming and everyone was doing exactly what they were supposed to be doing. I really do have an outstanding crew and I can't wait to be back there with them on a regular basis. Thanks to Eileen and the rest of them for being so tremendous!!

But Friday I learned it will be a while before I can go back to work because my Saturday activity was very limited. Pain comes and goes. Most of the pain is simply controlled by Tylenol. I do splurge at bedtime and take the narcotic, but hope to wean myself off of that soon. I do walk daily and walk longer every day. I feel I sleep too much, but the body is in charge of that and I fall asleep any time the body wants. Nothing planned for this week. My brother-in-law has two tickets for the Tiger game on Wednesday, two rows behind the dugout. I realize I am not ready for that; I will cheer on the Bengals from my couch. Friday I will see Dr. Hafez; he will receive a bear hug from me. I am lining up my questions for him.

The strength of FAITH dominates my thinking today. Jeannie is so strong. From the time of the diagnosis, she knew there would be no problem removing the tumor. I was scared to death and worried. Jeannie was like Martha in today's Gospel, **knowing** that the Lord would raise Lazarus from the dead. I was Lazarus wrapped in the bandages. Dr. Hafez was the Healer, simply doing what he had to do. The rest of you were the onlookers and the ones providing the prayerful support. What a ride this has been, remind me not to buy any more tickets.

Theresa told me to enjoy a beautiful Sunday walk. Camille was pleased to hear about how smooth everything at Burger King was. She complimented their leadership. She knows relief in that area will only improve my healing. The neurons in the brain will be happy and send happy messages. Aunt May wished us a great Sunday Supper; too bad she lives in Kalamazoo, too far to join us. She feels that God lets me spread my wings a little only to knock me back a bit, but there is progress.

Monday, April 11th:

Frank Berge wrote a great reflection: '"The reflections that you penned these past days during recuperation remind me of St. Ignatius of Loyola. While recuperating from a leg injury, he discovered the Lord's love for him and began treasuring life in radical new ways. Your journey together, St. Chuck and St. Jeannie of Brownstown, during these days of illness and recovery, is transforming both of you ... insight about your lives; the precious character of realities and your relationships with family members, friends and others with whom you share life is in a sense re-creating both of you. Thank you for being receptive to the Lord's love for you during these days of recuperation." *I think that Frank gives me more credit than I deserve. Sainthood? Must be a pretty accommodating membership. I do treasure life in radical new ways. I do know that, going forward, I have to make more time for prayers and meditation.*

Jane Paris enjoyed that reflection from me and the one from Frank. Jane thinks that the fact I think the progress is slow is a good sign. She read the following reflection in her beloved NCR: "In Ezechiel 37, we have the concept of resurrection in both its personal and communal sense and in its physical and spiritual sense. As I write, Lent is still a long way off. It is mid-October and the entombed coal miners in Chile are being lifted back to life in a capsule narrow enough to carry one man at a time through a tunnel drilled half a mile into the earth. Each wears sunglasses as protection from the coming onslaught of light. And, from above, as the capsule nearly reaches the surface, an orange-clad worker leans down and yells the miner's name. "Esteban" or "Claudio" or "Renan." When the miner calls back, the crowd, too, – workers, families, community leaders – chants his name and applauds, encouraging him to come from darkness back to life, from death back to life. Both the individual and community are resurrected, I cannot imagine hearing my name called from above, as the surface light begins to pierce the 70th day of my life in darkness. With that fierce determination I would call back, "Yes, here I am! It is me! I am alive!"

All I can say to that bone-chilling reflection is WOW!! It really hit home to me. Many times in my cancer journey I felt like I was in darkness and all of you jolted me back into life. This was culminated by the successful surgery almost three weeks ago. I have already expressed how useless TV has been during my recovery other than the Tigers. I do manage to watch CNN. This was one news story I closely followed. I was glued to the screen and watched many of those men be resurrected. My eyes were filled with tears of joy for complete strangers – they were my brothers!

Busted #2: I was filled with excitement after reading Frank's and Jane's words. They really lifted me up. One of the things I fill my time with is reading the Free Press. I have to bother others to get a copy of it, so I sometimes have to do without. Today was a day I was alone and had no source for the paper until after school. I wanted it NOW. As I am still unable to drive, I had to resort to the next best thing. My walks have been steadily improving so I thought I could make it to The Market for today's news. Off I went. I was nervous to be alone, but proud to be alone. It was my longest solo shot. WOOHOO! Mission accomplished! If only I had kept my mouth shut. No, I had to brag to the Warden. She launched into an unrepeatable diatribe about what she called an unrealistic decision. But I wasn't gonna let her rain on my parade, so I just smiled inside.

Tuesday, April 12th:

Today was my three-week anniversary of being cancer-free.

What a roller coaster ride 2011 has been. I have laughed a lot and I have cried a lot. I am proud to be here today. To celebrate, I went to Gabriel Richard for Mass. I was there three weeks ago on the way to surgery, so I felt it was only fitting to be there today. I wrote a letter to all of the students and staff thanking them for their support. I ended the letter by saying, "Prayer does work. Try it!" How many kids do not have time/room in their lives for God and prayer? Make the time! In his homily Fr. Bob talked about the need to spend more time expressing gratitude and less time expressing disappointment. That is a great challenge for me. How often do we ask God for help (daily for me) and how often do we thank God for what He has done for us (not nearly as often).

Also in today's entry I asked everyone to pray for Ryan's (my son-in-law's) grandma who is quite ill in Crittendon Hospital in Rochester. And I asked for prayers for Ryan and his family. All you have to do is ask. Many people wrote in the Guestbook and offered their prayers for his grandma and the family. We are all in this together.

Joy wrote in appreciating my three-week victory over cancer and said: "Sounds like God has certainly come across with Earl's request." Uncle Earl is not only one of my rocks, but Joy's as well. She, too, prayed to that dear man for his intercessions to Our Father. Mission Accomplished.

Chapter Eleven
A Spot on the Spine
The Rest of April

Friday, April 15th:

When we got home from the appointment at U of M, we found that there had been a power outage, and when the power surged back on, it blew up our beloved computer – a very important communication tool for me. What is worse is that we had nothing backed up. It is really a minor detail compared to cancer!

Before I saw Dr. Hafez, he sent in one of the resident interns. I do not remember if he was with me while I was in the hospital, but he was there today. He was pleased with the progress and told me not to be concerned with the remaining pain and numbness. This too shall pass. He had explained that they had to cut through four different sets of muscles and the recovery from that alone will be several months. Not what I wanted to hear, but it is what it is. He had no concerns with anything else, said I was a great healer.

The last part of the visit today dealt with a different concern. When I had the original CT scan in February, the scan showed a spot on the lower part of the spine. The docs all agreed to deal with the cancer first and then the silly spot later. Well the time is now. Jeannie brought it up to the young (they are quite young!) intern. He could not offer an instant answer. He left the room to confer with Dr. Hafez. They concurred that the spot is one of two things: It is either arthritis (please pray for arthritis) or there is a chance that the spot could be cancer – there goes that dreaded word again. Dr. Hafez was concerned as to whether or not I was physically and mentally ready for the testing due to the proximity of my surgery. I quickly said that I was ready and Jeannie agreed. Dr. Hafez and the intern looked at each other; made me wonder what they said when they were out of the room. The next step is that I will return to U of M, as soon as possible, for a biopsy and then they will be able to determine if I have the Big A or the Big

C. If it is cancer Dr. Hafez will refer me to a different oncologist who specializes with the spine. It is too early to tell what the treatment would be. Please pray for arthritis (I may have already said that.)

Monday, April 18th:

Once again I am amazed at the volume of support I received over the weekend. After all of the support since February 16th, why should I be amazed? It does feel good. This past weekend was anxiety-filled with the concerns about that damned spot, but we'll get through it, whatever the spot is. Wasn't there a Shakespeare play that had a line "Out, out, damned spot?" The phone calls, CB entries, emails, cards, text messages all lift me up when I am weak.

I did wish everyone a Happy Easter because I did not know how much I could get on the computer due to technical problems. Hard to believe that Easter is less than a week away and there are two inches of snow on the ground.

Thought for the day: "How you feel is more important than anything else, and you control how you feel!"

Tuesday, April 19th: Received a call from U of M and they have an opening on Thursday. Hooray! Very quick. It helps to relieve the anxiety. No time to worry. It is all done outpatient. No eating the night before, simple test (for them), and then I have to lay there for several hours of observation. Due to the Easter Holiday, they will not have the result until the following Tuesday at the earliest.

When I returned home, I was confused and nervous. In my heart, I knew God was with me and would continue to watch over me. What the heck, we have already beaten the Beast once this year – so bring it on. On the other hand I am human and mutter, "What if?" So I used the best resource I knew of: 1-800-Sr. Betty. I do not call her that often; and it amazes me that when I do need her, she answers the phone. She listened to me express my dilemma. When I was done blabbering, she made a startling revelation. She reminded me that we are in Holy Week and that I should compare and contrast my walk with the walk of Jesus. Another WOW moment. It truly helped me to understand the manifestation of God. And I was at peace. Now it is a short wait until Thursday.

The usual cast of characters weighed in on CB, offering their support during these few challenging days. Bev Beltramo laughingly commented, "Did you ever think you would be praying for arthritis?" The Jaskulas plan to offer their Easter Mass for me and extended the blessings of Christ's resurrection to me. Theresa is praying that the bump in the road will straighten out. Gwen is sending positive energy from Cleveland. Jim Vibbart reminded me that God IS good all of the time! – the repetition of the first words in Fr. Rick's homily at Ellen and Ryan's wedding.

Wednesday, April 20th:

I thanked our friend, Jeannette, as our pc is still dead, so we are writing due to the kindness of our loved ones. Tomorrow is the biopsy at U of M. Glad they got us in so quickly as I hate waiting, and this outcome is dominating my life. I asked everyone to pray hard for arthritis. I jokingly refer to it as Uncle Arthur, which reminds all of us of our dear next door neighbor and great Friend, Art Ford, who passed away at 96. I am sure learning lots about patience. By the time this is all over, I should have a Masters in Patience (MP).

Fr. Rick, in his Sunday homily, asked if we ever had one of those days where everything went wrong. I thought to myself that this whole year could fit that billing. Jesus had one of those days quite often during Holy Week. And the response of Jesus was, "Glory to God!" Quite an interesting response. Leave it to Jesus to challenge me when I don't want to be challenged. I think to myself, "Why me?" and Brother Steve said, "Why not you." So I have to start saying: "Why not me" and "Glory to God" a whole lot more.

Several good folks spoke on CB and they all said "Glory to God," it gets easier. Camille offered the following prayer: "May the good saints protect you and bless you. And may trouble ignore you each step of the way." She asked me to pray for her friend whose mother is waiting patiently for a heart transplant. Happy to do it. There are always those who need more prayers than I do. Glory to God!

Thursday, April 21st:

Biopsy Day. Another night of fasting – guess I am getting used to it. Another long questionnaire to fill out – guess I am getting used to it. The actual test was two hours late because the previous patient had an emergency – a stroke. The staff could not have been more apologetic. My logic is that if I had a stroke, I would have liked to be put to the head of the line as well. When I got to the Operating Room, the doc was exhausted due to the prior procedure. I asked if he wanted to freshen up before starting on me. He assured me he was fine and he was ready to go. They had to insert two needles through my back to withdraw the samples. The back bones are extremely strong and so they literally use a hammer to pound the needles into the back. Due to local numbing, I felt no pain. I could feel a continual rapid Tap, tap, tap, which was disconcerting. They took six or seven samples that will be analyzed by a pathologist. Tuesday is the earliest for the results.

My pain continues to lessen. Most of the time I can control it with Tylenol; there are rare times that I still need the narcotic.

There are lots of parallels in my life to walking with the Lord during this Easter week. Tonight's liturgy is my most favorite of the year. And the most symbolic feature is the washing of the feet. I need to wash all of your feet because of what you have done for me, by walking with me. At our church tonight, all of the youth going to see the Pope for World Youth Day had their feet washed by Fr. Rick. When Rick was done, he invited anyone from the congregation to come forward. I was so proud of Matthew; he went and washed the feet of a person that he had a disagreement with months earlier. They both cried – it was so moving. Simon helped Jesus to carry the cross – all of you are my Simons. The guard lanced the side of Jesus – I bet it looks like my side. Jesus endured what He did because the Father willed it. This cancer walk is not my choice, but I am enduring it with all of my "Simons." Thank You.

Friday, April 22nd:

Jeannie and I journey to St. Bonaventure Monastery for the first time. I will deal with this issue more at length in the next chapter.

Bev wrote that I have been doing the Good Friday walk these last two months. She thanked me for living the miracle and finding strength, courage, and faith to do what I had to do. She actually called me so strong. I get the strength from all of you.

Holy Saturday was so special. We began the day with a trip to the Eastern Market. I have been longing to go down there. We love to go to Vivio's for breakfast with our favorite waitress, Shirley. Then we browse through the vendor's stands looking for some awesome produce. The finale of the trip is a walk to the Rocky Peanut Company where Matt buys more candy than he needs. In Matt's absence, Jeannie does a fine job. By the time we got to Rocky's, my stamina was shot. I was happily eyeing the picnic table out front to sit down as this was my longest outing to date. I looked up and who was leaning against the building? Mike Meyers. His whole family, two kids and their significant others, his sister and her hubbie and his brother were all there. We have been friends for 40+ years, so this was a real treat and what a way to start the Easter Vigil. It was especially amazing to see Dani Meyers – the Lord has challenged her with many physical difficulties and she is in the process of winning. Through it all she has been so positive. I am so proud of her and gosh it was good to see her.

Even though the liturgy is over three hours long, it is an awesome three hours. What made it special is that Jeannie, Matt, and I were asked to do a three part reading. I was worried if I would be strong enough to do it, but it went off without a hitch. I am still weak and sit a lot in church, but I am there. After communion Deacon Mark approached me and wanted to know if I was all right. He had no knowledge of my cancer walk – now we have the newest member of the family.

Easter Sunday and Monday were very quiet. Lots of good will messages. Frank Berge is waiting for the Proclamation of more Good news on Tuesday. Another new family member today is Karen Pease, praying like the rest.

Tuesday, April 26th:

TIME TO CELEBRATE!! NO MORE CANCER!! THANK YOU JESUS!! What a relief it is. We have been anxious since the biopsy last Thursday. When the call came in around 12:45 PM, I naturally checked caller ID. I saw that it was U of M and I said to Jeannie, "Here we go!" The nurse was extremely professional and told me the results were negative. I started yelling, pumping my fist, and screaming for joy. I don't even remember ending the call. Our fervent prayers were answered.

The power of prayer. Still praying for Cyndi's mom, my second cousin, Kathy, thanking God for helping Ryan to get a new job, praying for Bill Rigg's parents. Each of you could go on and on. And now the Warden will only have one role in her life, to be my loving wife – who never stopped loving and has worked non-stop the last two months – really the last thirty two years. I AM BLESSED BECAUSE OF ALL OF YOU and still full of tears.

Chuck and Jeannie

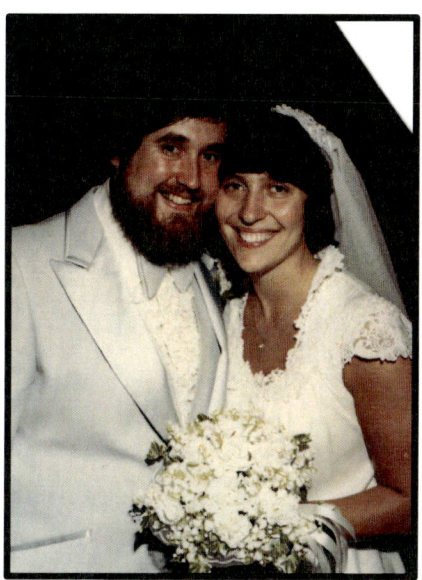

Wedding day
August 24, 1979

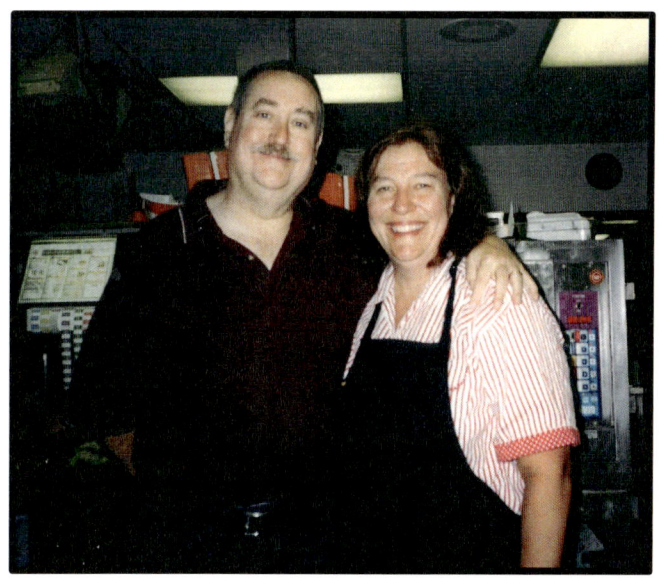

At Burger King
2010

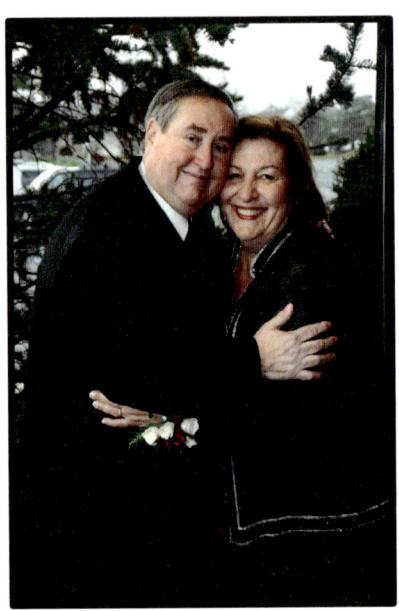

At Ellen's wedding
November 19, 2010

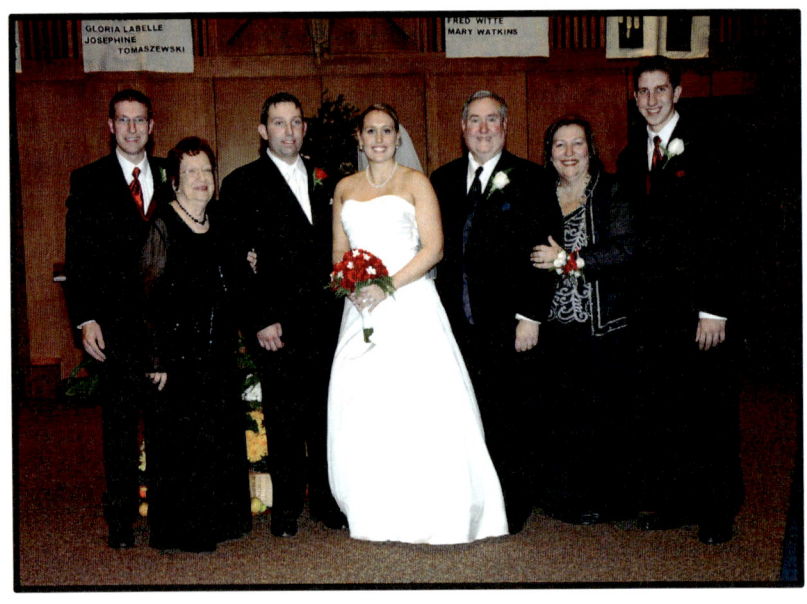

Piotrowski family at Ellen's wedding
November 19, 2010

Chapter Twelve

Walking with Barb Harrison, Solanus Casey, and Rita Late April and Early May

Early on in my cancer walk, I was invited to add Solanus to my walk. He did phenomenal things here in Detroit, mostly on the lower Eastside. The monastery on Mt. Elliott was his home. From what I have read, he truly is a Saint. In fact, early on, Sr. Mary Finn wrote to me and told me that Solanus needs one more miracle to receive the esteemed status of sainthood. She figures I should be the one to put him over the top. In fact, every time I see Sr. Mary she refers to me as a "miracle." Not that Sainthood was ever his goal. His followers, though, have worked hard to bring that lofty goal into reality. In this cancer walk, three different people have sent me a relic of his. I carry one with me in my wallet, one is in the dresser drawer next to my bed, and one is upstairs in my desk drawer. He is with me always. A recent visit with my friends Tom and Lorna DeGalen had Tom showing me his relic of Solanus in his wallet. A number of folks have also sent emails about Solanus and others have sent me Mass intention cards from his Guild. He is my 'GO TO" guy.

On Holy Thursday I received an incredible email from our dear friend Cyndi Harrison Popp. We worked with Cyndi in the late 70's at the SVdP camps. She was tremendously spirited and supportive lady. My favorite story about Cyndi focuses on how she would do anything for those camps. She received a prank phone call from one of us. The call announced that Camp Stapleton was selected at random by a fictitious radio station to receive a stereo. There was only one stipulation. Somebody from the camp had to drive through Port Sanilac with their car windows down while screaming, "We Love you Port Sanilac!" Once the call was placed, we scurried to town to hide behind some bushes to watch and laugh. It didn't take long, into town she and some others came, honking their horn, and screaming that phrase which I can hear loud and clear right now. They drove around screaming and didn't know what to do to claim their prize as the mysterious phone caller left out that detail. Finally we jumped out of the bushes as they drove past and laughed. What a prank.

Cyndi's email on Holy Thursday, April 21st, was also very passionate. It spoke about a mom's love for life and a daughter's love for her mom. She wrote: "Dear Friends, As most of you are aware, last April my mother was diagnosed with stage IV lung cancer. The months since then have been a blessing to me as we have shared memories and heartfelt exchanges. All those months since, she has continued to live independently in the home she loved. I was comforted with the virtual support of lifeline, and her sister who lives next door. She gave up driving in late June when she learned a tumor threatened to break her left hip. Her condition worsened within the last few weeks. She lost her appetite, has difficulty swallowing fluid, and is extremely fatigued. She is losing weight rapidly and growing weaker. Her wishes were for hospice palliative care. Today she went to Evangelica Nursing Home to spend her final days, until our great and merciful God calls her to her eternal resting place in Heaven. She is incredibly at peace, pain free and as amicable as ever. I would appreciate your prayers for her during her final days. Early on we went to Mass at St. Bonaventure. With individual special intentions she requested, "Grace filled and peaceful death." Won't you, too, join us in her special prayer intention?"

What an amazing prayer!! It really hit home to Jeannie and I for several reasons. Neither of us have ever met Barb, but we know and love Cyndi. Barb is preparing her death due to the same disease which I just had cut out of my body. And Barb, too, has a tie in to Solanus – too coincidental. We were on board with Cyndi's request – we would walk with Barb and Cyndi as long as they needed us. We were proud to be members of her prayer team. We would support the two of them and the family through our prayers and frequent emails.

The next day was Good Friday. Usually I am at Burger King

working during those special three hours. They may hold to be Christians, but we typically sell more Double Whoppers during those three hours than during any other three hours in the month. I am not sure why, it is just one of those eerie facts.

Our plan was to go to Our Lady of the Woods. After hearing from Cyndi, we immediately knew that we would make our first trip to the monastery. From the outside, it is not the most inviting place. We were not sure where to park and which door to use. As I tend to be early, there were no other cars around to guide us. We made a guess and entered a whole new world.

One is instantly filled with peace. The place is immaculately clean. We were immediately drawn to an area where sculpted statues are erected to modern day saints; the likes of Monsignor Clement Kern, Martin Luther King Jr., Mother Theresa, Dorothy Day, Jean Donovan, Archbishop Oscar Romero and Takashi Nagai. We felt so holy walking among these saints. There is a book store, selling many religious articles, informational literature about Solanus, and many other artifacts.

We now slowly made our way to the church itself. People were milling about and so we stepped back to observe what was going on. It didn't take us long to realize that, at the doors to the church, lay Solanus's crypt. What a holy spot. Against the walls people are able to sign in with their contact information and also sign in with their prayer intentions. Another outlet for their prayer intentions is to write them on a provided slip of paper, fold the paper in half, and then place the intention on his dear crypt. Once we figured out the routine, it didn't take me long to grab a pen and paper. I wrote two messages. The first one was to thank Solanus for walking with me in my cancer walk. The second one was that he walk with Barb and help her to achieve a "grace filled and peaceful death." I was in awe as I placed that slip of paper on that blessed crypt.

For the next three hours, we participated in a traditional Good Friday service. Good Friday was different for me this year. It had a deeper meaning and was much more prayerful. It is a small world, as one of the readers was Russ LeBlanc, whose late wife Pat worked with me years ago at St. Vincent de Paul.

I knew I found a new home that day and cannot wait to get back there. *Jeannie and I have decided to make an annual pilgrimage to the monastery on Good Friday as it was such a prayerful and moving experience. In 2012 we are going with Cyndi, our friend Bonnie and Bonnie's friend Kathy – who is struggling with her cancer. Solanus will help.* I look forward to a tour and getting to know those surroundings much better. I reflected back to Camp Ozanam days. Bernie Conway was the Camp Chairman. Any food that was left at the end of the summer that would not make it through the long winters was placed on a truck and driven down to the Capuchins and their Soup Kitchen. I guess Solanus has been in my life for quite a while.

I wrote about Barb on CB and instantly had a comment from Camille. She, too, was happy to hear that we were at the "site of dear Fr. Solanus. I have left many a written message on that very same spot. Even though you may feel weak-kneed and heart fain at times, I know your faith will pull you through." So Camille, too, walked with Barb.

We wrote to Cyndi and assured her of our support. We praised her for setting out to honor her mom's wishes. I told Cyndi that I would pray a rosary daily for her mom. In fact, while I was undergoing the bone scan of the spine on Holy Thursday last week, I figured would be an appropriate time. I did not have the beads, but I knew I could just use my fingers and count to ten. As I was continually rubbing each digit, one of the nurses viewed this process. He had no idea what I was doing, but he interpreted it that I was in pain and squeezing my fingers. He instantly ran over and began rubbing my shoulders to relax me. Not bad, I am getting a bone scan, praying the rosary, and receiving a massage all at the same time.

When we got home from the biopsy, there was an email waiting for us from Cyndi. "I'm incredibly touched (with tears) and appreciative of you offering a rosary for my mother during her final days. I, too, take comfort saying the rosary during other times of struggles. You are an amazing testament to our faith, always putting others before your own needs… I am praying that your biopsy results represent good news!" *It is with humility that I even include this quote. All God ever asks of us is to do what we can. Walking with Barb and Cyndi during those days was easy. It is what we needed to do. Besides, a little diversion is always good.*

We then called our daughter, Ellen, and shared with her our moving story about going to the monastery. We shared with her the awesome details about visiting the crypt and leaving our intentions safely with Solanus. Ellen stopped me and said, "Dad, I know. I've been there and it works!" Wow! I was assured right then and there that the biopsy results would be negative. I asked Ellen to explain how she knew that. Ellen explained that she was there in the spring with her fourth grade class from St. Stephen's. She too wrote down an intention and placed it on that holy crypt. I asked her if she minded sharing with me what she wrote about. She explained that her older brother was going through some tough times and she asked Solanus to walk with Joe. How awesome is that – Ellen praying for her brother. That's what family is all about. And the best part is that her prayers worked and Joe is in a much better place today than he was beforehand.

Wednesday, April 27th:

Cyndi added to the list of people rejoicing over my biopsy results. Here again is another testament to the faith that Cyndi wrote about earlier. Her mom is clinging to the last days of her life, but Cyndi had time for us. Cyndi shared my special Easter prayer journey with her mom who teared up and nodded approvingly about my shared prayer intention with Fr. Solanus. Cyndi said: "She is still at peace and not in any pain. I remain steadfast in honoring her wishes. She gave me a mini refresher course earlier. Thanks for your and Jeannie's support. It is very uplifting!" *WE LIFT UP EACH OTHER!*

Friday, April 29th:

I wrote to Cyndi after watching the fairy tale wedding of William and Kate. Jeannie and I did not have quite that elaborate of a ceremony, but it was just as exciting as the one on TV, if not more. And I am sure the same is true for Cyndi and Steve. I then mentioned to Cyndi about the existence of the Caring Bridge website and suggested she might look at it.

I went on to explain that one of the most recent hits on the website was from our friend Theresa Howard. She commented that Fr. Solanus regularly visited her grandfather's farm to pick up food to deliver to the poor. Is that awesome? And Fr. Solanus cured Theresa's grandfather of cancer. Their family name (Eagen) is often mentioned in biographies of Fr. Solanus.

Cyndi responded later in the day and did visit the CB website. She again humbled me by saying, "What a moving and honest journal of a great couple so strong in faith – travelling along life's uncertain roads. I am rejoicing with you all at your great news. You and Jeannie will forever be remembered in all my future Easter petitions of thanks for the compassion and support you have given Barb and I during our final Easter together. My mom deteriorated very quickly. She recognized me a few days ago and is happy I am with her – I asked her if she wanted me to stay and she nodded yes. I moved in two days ago. Sadly the pain kicked in last night. Very rough to witness and try to help her get situated to get comfortable. She crosses herself nonstop when she's uncomfortable. Please pray that our Merciful Loving God carries her home to rest soon, (with tears flowing)" With *tears flowing is an interesting way for Cyndi to end this entry. I can surly identify with that. I have cried more in 2011 than I did in the previous 58 years. There is nothing wrong with freely expressing emotion. The tears often say more than words could ever hope to.*

In this entry Cyndi referred to her mom unconsciously crossing herself when she was uncomfortable. Women of faith do that. An example of this is my mother-in-law, Jeanne Byron aka Nonnie. A while ago she was in Mercy Memorial Hospital in Monroe. She went through a rough spell and was not conscious. What did she do? Repeatedly said the Our Father, the Hail Mary, prayed for the poor souls in purgatory and crossed herself. The crossing of one's self is really a blessing! Also amazing is how strong Barb and Nonnie's faith is that even in an unconscious state they pray. What an awesome witness these women are.

Walking with Solanus is amazing and healing. Our friends, Mike and Kathy Morris emailed today. They have a friend that received a donation request from the Monastery and so they decided to take a field trip to the Monastery. Cathy figures we were there at the same time on Good Friday. Wow! The lady who went to the monastery that day had a great grandmother-in-law who lived to be 107 years old and drank a shot of holy water daily. The lady's father-in-law is following the same routine along with a new medicine designed to shrink the cancer cells to keep them from growing larger.

Cathy then wrote, "I will be going to see Noelle Mann, my niece who just had a baby boy, Milo William, at 6:27 today. He is 7lb. 5oz., and 20 inches long. The Lord giveth and the Lord taketh away." *How profound and how true that is so many times in life.*

Saturday, April 30th:

When I woke up this morning, I checked my emails. There were a couple brief ones from Cyndi saying that the end was definitely near.

Cyndi wrote to her support group: "I am immeasurably grateful to each of you for answering my prayer plea for my mother, Barbara Harrison. I heard from each of you and felt your uplifting comfort and support. How blessed I am. Imagine if you will a very quiet room with soft church hymns playing. (With the wonders of technology I built a "Hospice" playlist for my IPhone that included a variety of soothing music.) Mother was resting comfortably when, at approximately 4:00 AM, a change in her breathing took place. One of the many nurse angels, Dorothy, confirmed that her final hour was nearing. I was able to call in our small immediate family to join her bedside for our final goodbyes. This morning at 8:50 AM my Mother, in the most peaceful beautifully imaginable way, departed this earth to join her Shepherd, our Lord. I remembered at the very end this was her favorite verse: The Lord is My Shepherd. Years ago I cross stitched this verse with the depiction of a shepherd tending his flock in a field for her. This was hung in her bedroom at her prayer station. While I was gently imploring her to follow her Shepherd, our favorite hymn, **Be Not Afraid,** was playing. That is when she drew her last breath. Not so much as a grimace crossed her face. Her complexion was perfect and her hair looked beautiful as always. I will greatly miss my mother's unconditional love and support. I hope each of you get to experience the peace and tranquility of helping a loved one transition from this life into God's paradise." Wow – what a eulogy. Cyndi could take up writing as well.

The interesting thing here is that I never met Barb and really don't see Cyndi that often, but when we got the email that Barb had passed I cried like a baby. It is a great feeling to walk the last few days of someone's life with them. So her death, her wish, was a bit of a letdown as well.

Barb's wish at the end helped me to reflect on my mom's passing in 2004. Rita wanted to die in her own home. She had been in a nursing home since July. At the end of August it was obvious her time was near, so we took her home to 10th Street, her wish was fulfilled.

That last week was so special. My family was pleased to walk with her. We were blessed to have her guardian angel, Nadine, be with her when we were unable. She slept a lot and ate very little. At the time of her death she weighed 78 pounds.

Two days before she died, she was hungry – we were all surprised. She had to have a banana split. So we went and got her dear friend, Helen Sarnacki, to join us. It was her farewell party, as she never ate again. (In her honor, Crystal Gardens served banana splits at her funeral luncheon. I lost count as to how many our long-time friend Stanley consumed.)

The night before mom died we gathered around her bed. She was unconscious and thrashing around. We did not have a clue if she was even aware of our presence. Joe reached out and tickled her right foot. One of Rita's pet peeves is to have anyone touch her feet. Even I was appalled with Joe's unwanted gesture. To my surprise, as Joe touched her foot, she stopped thrashing and smiled. In a deep, barely audible voice she said. "Hi Joe!" She knew that only Joe would be bold enough to touch her foot and was aware of our presence. "Hi Joe" were the last words she uttered.

The next day she peacefully passed away with her guardian angel softly singing a hymn in her ear. Her funeral, like Barb's, was a true celebration of her life. Most days in the nursing home and especially those last six days on 10th street, I ended my visit with my mom by tracing the sign of the cross on her forehead and saying, "God Bless you and keep you safe." At her funeral, the assembly was invited to do that to each other at the Kiss of Peace – quite a gesture. It is a gesture that I continue to use as I visit the patients at Southshore.

Tuesday, May 3:

Due to a prior commitment, Jeannie and I were unable to attend Barb's funeral. Truth be told, we were in Las Vegas at a Burger King convention (more about that in the next chapter). We did pray with Cyndi and her family that day. Probably one of the few rosaries prayed from Sin City. Cyndi wrote to us and shared the highlights from the liturgy. She included the songs, the readings, and even her tribute. It was like we were there. Cyndi was lifted by her mom during the tribute; no tears. Barb's trust bequeathed $10,000 to the Solanus Casey Center. Throughout the wake, folks donated another $600 and I know other donations came in after that. What a noble way to remember somebody. Cyndi thanked us for being her special angels. It was a pleasure, my dear.

As a PS, she included her mother's favorite Lotto numbers. She suggests betting 35 in her mom's honor; might be worth a shot.

Saturday, May 7:

At 9 a.m. today was Barb's committal ceremony at Resurrection Cemetery. The setting was incredible, as all of the trees were in full bloom. As Cyndi walked to her car, she spotted the biggest blue jay, perched on a flowering branch. What a peaceful sight. The blue jay story reminded me again of my mom. When Rita came home for those last days, she wanted her flowering beds cleaned up. Joe literally pulled up every plant by their roots and then raked the whole bed to get it ready for winter. Rita was pleased to have this work accomplished. We thought nothing more about it.

Saturday after Rita's memorial service, we returned to 10th Street. We were in awe because as we pulled up to the curb, there was one Lazy Susan in full bloom. It is totally impossible for that to have happened. It was my mom waving good-bye to us all. We all cried our final good-byes to her as well.

Chapter Thirteen

Beginning to Return to Normalcy
April 26– May 7

Tuesday, April 26:

(Took a slight diversion from the chronological story to tell Chapter 12.) Once the news got out that the spine biopsy was negative, the CB network exploded. Karen Pease was a new signer. Frank Berge did the best summary when he exclaimed, "Basking in the glory of it all!" Gregg Shields invited me for a weekend to Dallas to celebrate. Jim Vibbart celebrated with a cup of "joe" which he bought at his favorite Burger King – mine!

Wednesday, April 27:

The positive stuff on CB continued. Joy and Anne both used the same word, "Alleluia" – seems pretty appropriate to me. Aunt May commented that my recovery continues with a happy heart.

Sr. Marge wrote an awesome entry. I feel like I have known this woman for years and it is only four months. I actually called her with the news. She talked about how powerful the prayer connections are within my support group, which is larger than I ever imagined. "May God continue to bless and support you as you are surrounded by so many caring people."

The interesting thing about this interlude with the spine biopsy is that in Jeannie's mind it was never something to be concerned about. I was sitting on pins and needles. My faith told me all would be well. My mind drifted to the "what if?" stage. "What if?" is a horribly negative term. It should be struck from my vocabulary. Even if the biopsy had been cancerous, I would have reached out to my God and all of you and successfully dealt with it. It is easy to say now – not so easy to say a few weeks ago.

Friday, April 29th:

A very interesting day for me. I was contacted by one of the students from Gabriel Richard. As you are aware, the GR community has walked with me throughout this cancer journey. They are incredible. Now they want a favor from me. Now it's time for me to give back to them. They are involved in the Riverview Relay for Life. They have asked me to participate. Wow!! It is indeed my pleasure to say yes. As a cancer survivor I am allowed to walk the first lap. I will not be out to set any speed goals, but I am proud to be a part of the GR team.

I also learned today that my sister and her family will be participating in a 100 mile bike ride to benefit cancer research and she is dedicating her ride in my honor – it takes your breath away. All of that for me. Wow!

I commented that I do feel better each day and that sometimes borders on cockiness – how far can I push the envelope. There are more good days than bad. Today I thought of my favorite paraphrased quotes from one of my favorite motivational speakers, Zig Ziglar: "You can have anything you want, as long as you help someone else get what they want." That is so true.

Saturday, April 30th:

This was the date of death of two people for whom I have asked all of my CB buddies to pray. The first one was Barb Harrison, to whom the last chapter was dedicated. The second one was Ryan's (my favorite son-in-law) grandmother. Grandma had not been in the best of health. She came to Michigan to try and improve her situation, but there was no strength in her body. May they both rest in peace.

Once again people's kindness was witnessed by me today. I mentioned in yesterday's CB posting that I was asked to do the Relay for Life Walk and today Anne and Paul want to know where to send their donation. Wow! Thanks guys!

Sunday, May 1:

"Wherever you go, there you are." There is no such thing as being anonymous. It is a small world. We landed in Vegas and were waiting at the carousel for our luggage. Some large packages rode past us, much larger than normal. We wondered out loud, whose they were and what they contained. It didn't take long to get an answer. There, on the other side of the conveyor, stood our friend, JR Freiburger. He was exhibiting at the Burger King convention and was getting all his props. JR and Connie have been frequent visitors to CB. It was thrilling to see him and he gave us one of the warmest embraces you can imagine.

Monday, May 2nd:

Matt's 17th birthday. My baby is growing up. He has never been a baby – too darn big! He has inherited his brother's ability to be positive. I recognize Matt for being a well-rounded individual. Academically his GPA is probably double the one I achieved. He plays two sports. He has a great faith life. He is involved in many extracurricular activities at his beloved GR. Yes, we have our run-ins -- after all, he is a teenager. There is not a day that goes by that he does not look at his mom and I in which he hugs us and says, "I love you." That is so special that he is not afraid to express his love, and then demonstrate it. I love you Matt.

Jeannie and I had pre-registered for the BK convention before we learned of the cancer, otherwise we might not have gone. Since the trip was paid for we decided to go for it. Jeannie is always a planner and thoughtful. She made arrangements for a wheel chair for me everywhere we went. I didn't want one, but you don't argue with The Warden. Using hindsight, it was definitely helpful in the airport, with the long walks in between terminals. Could I have made it without a wheel chair? We'll never know. It was extremely helpful with boarding the airplanes. First on and first off. And we sat in the first row with the extra leg room. That was nice! Pride and dignity kept me from using the wheel chair in the hotel during the actual convention – I didn't want to be seen as an invalid. May not have been my wisest decision, but we went with it. I can tell you this, by the end of the convention I was more exhausted than I have ever been - so much for pride.

Walking around visiting the vendors is always fun. Yes, they are all trying to sell a product, but we are all humans with our own stories to tell. At one booth (Maines Paper), the gentleman and I exchanged our cancer stories as we are both cancer survivors. He asked me how I would describe how cancer changed my life. What a succinct question. I thought for a moment and then I said that it changed me in two ways: 1. It has made me much more emotional. I cry a lot. I guess I have always been somewhat sentimental, but I am ten times worse. The emotions can be happy or sad events. If it has an impact on my life, I cry! Being emotional is not necessarily a manly trait, but who cares. It is one that I own and I am proud of it. Cancer has helped me to appreciate the moment and to freely express it. I am blessed!

2. Cancer has greatly deepened my relationship with the Lord. I used to pray when it was convenient and when I made the time for it – never as much as I should have. Now my day is filled with much more prayer. Before my feet hit the floor, I thank God for the gift of another day. I thoroughly enjoy talking daily with God! I still struggle with writing in that Gratitude Journal, but I am better at it. I have so much to be grateful for, and so much family and friends to praise. The new found devotion to the rosary is enjoyable. Many nights when my brain thinks too much and I can't sleep, I employ those beads and pray for whoever is dominating my thoughts.

Our son, Joe, lives in Vegas and while we were there I shared with him the above two observations. He got kind of quiet and said, "Geesh, dad, I always thought you had a great faith relationship with the Lord. It makes me wonder, what does mine look like?" I told Joe that only he can answer that question. If he is not happy with the answer then it is up to him to do something about it. Joe is of the generation (I am sure there is a name for his generation) that questions their faith a lot. It is not fulfilling enough to go to the church of their childhood. They are searching. In Joe's case I challenge him about his faith life, a lot! It is not only about going to church on Sunday, but it is a great place to start. (I wonder what Joe's comments will be when he reads this – no sneak previews). Joe has some concerns about the Catholic faith. That's fine. What other avenue will he follow? Don't tell me how hard you work all week and that Sunday is your day to sleep in. Crap!! I don't care where you go to worship, just go and Praise the

Lord! (enough of the soap box).

Thursday, May 5th:

We got home from Vegas and we were pooped. My head could not hit the pillow fast enough. Of course, when we hit the door, we had to skim the mail and listen to voice mail. I found it curious that I had three voice mails from U of M – what could they want? It was 9:00 PM and so my question could not be answered until the morning.

Friday, May 6th: I couldn't dial U of M fast enough; curiosity was killing this cat. When I finally reached the nurse she explained that she was calling me with the results from the biopsy that was taken on April 22nd. I told her that I had been given those results by a kindly woman on April 26th. I told her that I knew I was going to be out of town so I was a tad pushy because I knew I would enjoy my trip more knowing what the results were. The woman got extremely quiet. I asked her if there was a problem. She said she was rereading all of the notes. Due to the Easter Holiday, there was a delay in receiving the test results. The results did not come back until April 29th. Furthermore, the meticulous notes which U of M keeps to make sure that they all know what each other is doing, did not indicate that anyone had called me. She said, "WITH ALL RESPECT, SIR, IT IS IMPOSSIBLE THAT ANYONE CALLED YOU ON THAT TUESDAY, and THE RESULTS WERE NOT AVAILABLE THAT EARLY!" We both were quiet. Who called? We will never know, but you will never convince me that the Lord did not have a hand in this. That phone call eased the pressure and did help me to enjoy Las Vegas all the more. Many times I have wondered if it wasn't U of M, who was it? The caller ID identified the first call as U of M. I clearly was being carried in the palm of Jesus!!!

On Saturday, May 7th, I wrote my last journal entry on Caring Bridge-- what a powerful tool that website had been. We all walked together with a few pecks on the key board. TR wanted to know what I would do with my free time, if I wasn't going to use Caring Bridge anymore. I told Brother T that I have grown fond of using this form of communication, so I would now stick to the key board and write a book about my cancer experience. "We Beat the Beast" is the proposed title of the book. My entire support group will be the co-writers as all of them/you have walked every step with me. Now that I have announced this, I have to do it. Too many folks will challenge me if I don't. I hope that my thoughts are worthy enough to be published. Through this cancer journey, TR has called me his hero. Can he really be that desperate? I just dealt with the hand of cards I was given and, surrounded by people filled with God's grace, we beat the beast.

Later that day many people called or emailed or Bcc'd (is that a real term?) to comment on my last entry. I am still amazed at how many people found my entries inspiring. I was certainly inspired and in awe of the wonderful support that I received from all of them/you. Aunt May said that: "Your trust in God, prayer, and friends have been outstanding. I am proud to say that I am related to you; because of you I too have been blessed. I will miss the updates that you have given us especially on the down days, which were hard to deal with as you wanted to move forward and couldn't." I guess the Caring Bridge was a small part of the daily lives of many.

Camille emailed that day. The friendship that I now have with Camille is so special because I have never met her. She wrote: "I am so happy to hear you are on the yellow brick road and looking into the daily sunrise without the stress of cancer. You have added joy, and have awakened awareness of the power of Faith. You did that for me! Perhaps one day our paths shall cross." *One of the happier days of the summer for me came in mid-June. Jeannie and I took Matthew for a tour of Kalamazoo College and Western. As both of those universities are near Nazareth, where Aunt May lives, we decided to surprise her and stop in for an unannounced visit – aren't surprises grand! It was unbelievable that Camille just happened to be visiting that week – so we finally got to meet. My new friend has a body and the warmest smile one can imagine!*

Our dear camp friend, Bonnie, was the last person to write in the Guestbook. She said that my ending of CB was a big Healing step. She challenged me to be patient. She vowed continued support and said, "YOU ARE NOT IN THIS ALONE!"

Chapter Fourteen
May Showers Bring...
The Rest of May

At the beginning of May, I received an email from our friend. Bonnie. Bonnie was able to be a strong support for Cyndi during her mom's walk. Bonnie said, "Shortly after getting back to work, and returning a phone call, I found out that another friend has cancer again!! She gets her port tomorrow and starts chemo the following week. I'm angry, upset!! She's been through it once and lost her husband to it after a long battle. She's scared and I told her we would be positive. So if you don't mind, can I ask you to add my friend, Kathy, to you prayers? Thank you. *It was a pleasure to add Kathy to my prayer list. I emailed Kathy that day and have continued to pray for her and her health (both mental and physical) for a few months now. We email back and forth. She has sent me a couple of very powerful prayers. Who's the patient here? Take a moment now and pray for Kathy or somebody you know who is the victim of this potentially ravishing disease. Thank You.*

I got another email from Bonnie the next day, apologizing for the above email. Bonnie was concerned that I am still in recovery and she is adding more work to my life. Prayer is never work; it is always a blessing. It is time for me to give back. Isn't that what life and family are all about? We all help each other, so it is my privilege to walk with Kathy.

On May 6th I was lucky enough to meet one of the newer members of my family, Marcella. She is the daughter of one of my crew members, Marsha. One of my managers also gave birth to a son, Noah, during my absence. Life goes on. More and more good people are welcomed into this wonderful world of ours.

On May 13th, Brother Steve was nice enough to drive me out to Burger King. I am getting stronger, but my stamina is just not what I wished it would be. When I got home from Burger King, I took advantage of the shade from a pear tree and slept in the back yard. I was pleasantly surprised by a phone call from Pat and Karla O'Grady. They were calling to offer their support. When I heard of their health struggles, it made my cancer walk seem like a stroll in the park. Pat humbled me with the following question: "Chuck, with all of the good things you have done for others, why did God give you cancer?" I do appreciate Pat recognizing my goodness, but I am not really that good. The short answer to that question was that "God can." He challenged me and all of you responded. Thank You!

On May 14th we had a shower at our home for Amy Owens, who is marrying our nephew, Pete. What an exciting time – makes me reflect back to the time of my engagement and dreaming of spending my life with Jeannie – if she knew then…

On May 17th I saw Dr. Nazareno. From his perspective, he thought it looked like everything was going well. I always go to the doctor without eating, just in case he wants to draw blood. I was right on today. Off I went to the clinic at Southshore. Unbelievably, the results were available the next day. Now that's service, folks. All of the results were very good, including the A1C count; it was the lowest it has been in three years. Wow!

When I got home from Dr. Nazareno's office, I had doctors on my mind. As you know from reading this book, I have the utmost respect and admiration for my doctors – especially Dr. Nazareno and Dr. Hafez. I see Dr. Nazareno often and express my gratitude directly to him. As I rarely see Dr. Hafez, I decided to write him a letter of thanksgiving. In the letter I praised him for his wisdom and support during my cancer journey. That support was highlighted by his phone call two days before my surgery. As I closed my letter, I told him about this very book. I promised him the very first copy. The only problem is I have promised the first copy to a lot of folks – not sure how I will get around that. Secretly, I was hoping to hear back from him. I am not sure why; it's not like he has the time to cultivate a friendship with me.

I just admire him tremendously and needed to tell him so.

On May 20th we travelled back to our second home, Ann Arbor. It is a slight inconvenience, but it is nice to have everything under one roof. We met with Dr. Wang, the gastro guy. As always, U of M updates their medical records before every visit. Through this process I have lost 35 pounds and am happy; I do not recommend the cancer diet though. As I got on the scale, we learned that I have gained almost 10 pounds – was I disgusted. Dr. Wang, on the other hand, was thrilled. He explained that was the most positive sign that the healing process has begun. In fact, he would have been very concerned if I had lost more weight. Never thought I would be happy to gain weight.

On May 20th we celebrated the life of Louie Collura, Coney Dave's dad. Louie was an awesome man, who never stopped giving. The night before, at the wake service, his family asked me to lead those gathered in a rosary. It is the first time I have ever been asked to do that. I was more than a little nervous, but was honored to do it. In each decade of the rosary I only prayed nine Hail Marys. Those who were following closely had puzzled looks on their faces. At the end of the rosary, I explained that I skipped one Hail Mary in each decade on purpose. The reason being that, when people remembered that I skipped those five Hail Marys, they could say them at that time in Louie's honor. The highlight of the funeral came when one of Louie's granddaughters sang a hymn in his honor. What a voice she had. The lyric that really struck a chord with me was when she said that earth is only "our temporary home." We often think of it as our permanent place, but it is our temporary home.

BUSTED #3 – I woke up on the morning of May 23rd feeling strong. I was a tad cocky. Jeannie diligently prepared me breakfast, as she has been doing all of these weeks. She then made my lunch and went off to GR. Today I would make my GREAT ESCAPE. She hadn't hid the garage door closer and I was up and getting dressed. I was going to Burger King ALONE. You cannot imagine my excitement. I figured if I was too tired I would just pull over and nap. I knew if I asked the Warden for a pass, it would be denied. Hi Ho Hi Ho – it's off to work I go. What a thrill! Everything went off without a hitch.

All was well in Whitmore Lake. I stayed for a short visit and drove home. I was careful to park the car exactly as I had found it. I went in the house and ate the previously prepared lunch. When Jeannie got home from GR, I was sleeping, like my routine. When I got up, I made no mention of my Great Escape. We were having normal conversation at the dinner table. I commented how excited I was to know that our monthly Speed of Service was under the demanded 2:30. DUH! Jeannie stopped and wanted to know how I knew that. I said that I looked it up online. Jeannie saw right through that line of hooey and I was busted, but it still felt good.

On May 24th I received an interesting letter from Max Wicha, the director of the Cancer Center at U of M. It was the most sincere fundraising letter I have ever received. He believes that we can win this War on Cancer. President Nixon signed the National Cancer Act over forty years ago. Mr. Wicha feels: "Between 1975 and 2007, the mortality rates for some of the most prevalent cancers declined by double digits. Five year survival rates for most cancers have increased markedly. But for many tumor types, and far too many cancer patients, outcomes have been far less promising. **Overall, our results are just not good enough.**" Mr. Wicha believes that we can win this war, but they need financial support to continue the fight. I know that the charity of supporting the war on cancer will move to the top of my list. At the end of the book I will provide contact information, if you are so inclined. We all support meaningful charities or we wouldn't be a part of the human race.

Three days later, on May 27th, Jeannie and I went to Burger King together. It is always good to go to Burger King. I have still not redeveloped a taste for any food. My diet is always oatmeal and peanut butter and jelly, with a few variations thrown in. I do not even have a craving for a Whopper. Our visit was ok. Unfortunately, I did not find everything running as smoothly as I thought it should be. I started challenging the staff. My patience got the best of me and I could feel my temperature rising. I knew I only had one option before I did more harm than good. I left and went to sit in the car. I did not say good bye. Half an hour later, Jeannie noticed I was missing and she found me sulking. The funny thing is that, as I write this, I do not have a clue as to what possessed me to walk out. I just knew whatever it was that was attacking me, I had to leave before I said or did something I would later regret.

BUSTED #4 – One of the things that relaxes me the most is a nice soaker in the tub. I had been told by the staff at U of M that I was only allowed to take showers. This exile to the shower stall was never meant to be permanent so I decided today was the day to broaden my horizons. I knew the Warden would not grant me permission, so I quietly made arrangements for my first dunk in the tub. I was afraid that the sound of running water might be my slip up, but there really is no quiet way to get water in the tub. The Warden did not catch me – Whew! However, her #1 deputy (Matthew) did. He heard the water running and looked at his mom and said, "What does he think he is doing?" With that he charged into the bathroom, put his hands on his hips, glared at the prisoner (poor little ole me), and said, "What do you think you are doing?" Having to answer to my baby is a little disconcerting. I asked him what did it look like I was doing? He just stood there and shook his head. He then queried, "How do you think you are going to get out of the tub?" I told him that was my problem and if I needed the big lunk's help I would call. It was a struggle to get out. One thing I learned that day, it would be a long time before I next tried to take another bath.

On May 30th, my cockiness gave me a bit of a physical set back at work. I was walking through the back room and noticed that a couple of soda pops needed to be changed. I glanced around and saw nobody nearby. What the heck, I have changed thousands of these over the years. So I proudly changed the pops. Ouch. Two problems, they get heavier as I get older and I had to reach over my head to replace a few. Mentally I was excited to do this, physically I was a wreck. It will be a long time before I attempt to do this again. If only I followed the Warden's directives….

Chapter Fifteen

... June Flowers
The Month of June

June 4th was the day I was waiting for, the city of Riverview's Relay for Life. It was a glorious day. TR and Barb were in town and decided to join us at the start. Unfortunately, the pre-event activities were moving too slowly for the always-moving couple so they left before the event kicked off. I did appreciate their support by being there. Jeannie, Ellen, and I joined together for this special day. Thankfully, we all brought sun glasses as the sun was shining the brightest it had all spring; how appropriate was that? We checked in at the GR booth. Then we checked in at Headquarters. I was given a sash to wear that bore the words "cancer survivor" and a pin stating the same to apply to the sash. It was a moving moment as Jeannie slipped that sash on me. On my head I wore the ever-present GR hat. As often as possible, I wear that hat or other apparel to promote that awesome institution. We approached the stage to listen to some speeches. A woman spoke of her husband's cancer journey. A little over five years ago, he was given six weeks to live. The villain cancer was hard at work. The couple prayed together and turned his care over to some awesome doctors. And now 5 1/2 years later he was on the stage. Alleluia! There wasn't a dry eye in the house! He spoke briefly and said, "It ain't over until God says it's over!" He stated that they prayed the day they received the diagnosis and decided that their number one goal each day is to start the day praising the Lord and thanking Him for the gift of another day -- a good challenge for me and all of you. After his remarks, his wife returned to the microphone and sang to her husband, telling him (and sharing that witness with all of us) that he was her hero.

Now it was the time for the main event. All of the cancer survivors were invited to walk the first lap. I knew I wanted to do a mile so the three of us set out to walk three laps. The course was around a pond. Standing around the pond were hundreds of concerned supporters, who applauded as we walked by. We walked with our head held high. Jeannie held my right hand and Ellen held my left; those two have literally been with me every step of the way. Thank God for those sunglasses as all three of us admitted to crying every step of the way (*I am shedding a couple of tears as I type this.*) I have not been that moved in a long time. I was proud to lead that walk and help Relay for Life in their fundraising endeavors.

June 5th brought about the conclusion of the Relay. Jeannie had decided we wanted to walk another supportive mile. We got there at 6:00 AM. There were only a few stalwart supporters left as the wee morning hours claimed some bodies. We saw this as a great opportunity to pick up the slack and proudly set off on our mile, still wearing those sunglasses. After one lap an announcement was made, asking for help with picking up the expired luminaries. At dusk last night, several hundred luminaries were placed around the course. Each luminary bore the name of a cancer survivor, a cancer victim, or of a supporter. Each luminary had a candle inside, many of which were still lit, over nine hours later. As the ranks of the supporters had dwindled, the task of picking up the luminaries was pretty daunting. It was very interesting to pick up a luminary and find the name of somebody we knew; time for a prayer for that person! As we stomped on the candles to put them out, we thought of the strength of prayer and research that together we would someday stomp out cancer. We were able to accomplish that mile and to do service by removing the luminaries. And we were able to pray for the eventual conquering of cancer.

Today is also Jeannie's birthday. All I can say is Wow! Can you imagine a more supportive human being? That is the quality of Jeannie's that I admire the most. And she has been supportive in the thirty five years I have known her; it goes beyond the cancer journey. Many spouses who read this could say the same thing about their own spouses, let's hope so! Jeannie though leads the pack! I love you, Jeannie.

I wanted to celebrate her birthday in a special way. In our calendar, I just wrote the word "surprise!" She hates surprises and kept bugging me for information. Being a last minute person, I had none. In the last few days, the details all fell together. We were going to the casino! In addition to trying our luck at the machines, we would spend the night and have dinner at Wolfgang Puck's, a restaurant that is managed by one of her former students- yup another GR graduate. After checking into our deluxe room, we went in search of our lucky machine. We found an unbelievable ally in a two-cent machine that just kept giving and giving. It was hard to believe that in less than an hour we were over $1,000 ahead. Now it was time for dinner. Jeannie was a little quiet as we approached the restaurant. I knew why and smiled sheepishly to myself. Birthdays are family affairs. She was loving the one-on-one time with me, but celebrating without her kids, was a tad disappointing. Imagine her joy, as she rounded the corner in the restaurant and she spotted Matt, Ellen, and Ryan waiting there for us. Wow! Wow! A short time later, Joe called right on cue. What a perfect two days those were. Happy Relay for Life and Happy Birthday.

On June 7th our dear friend, Jim Vedro, came over for dinner. Jim is a special man and was extremely supportive during the cancer journey. As he lives in Minnesota, we only see him once or twice a year. So tonight was the first time, since being cancer-free, that we have been together. It was great to see him and share a wonderful pork chop barbeque together. Jim's prayers and constant emails helped move me along.

June 8th: Happy Birthday Ellen. Two words summarize our darling daughter, intense and shoes. She owns more pair of shoes than any two women I know. If there is a sale she is on it. If there is a tall heel she is on it. If there is a flashy shoe she is on it. Her goal is to own a different pair for every day of the year. That alone is intense, but that same intensity spills into her everyday life. Whether she is teaching, doing the crossword in People, baking, watching the Bachelor, loving her hubby or many other things – she is intense. Wonder where she gets that from? All I know is when you are friends with Ellen, you get one of the strongest friendships you can imagine. She never stops giving. Happy Birthday, Ellen!

June 10th was another sad day. One of my classmates, Fr. Bill Lunnon was buried today. Bill has led a seemingly tormented life and he died way too young, but it was his time. The St. Cecilia choir sang some very moving spirituals. It was a great send-off for Bill. Mr. Guenther was in attendance and I remarked how weird it was to bury a classmate. He said it is even stranger to bury a former student. In Bill's honor, Ron Victor, Jeannie and I went to lunch at the Burger King nearest St. Cecilia's.

When I got home from the funeral there was an email from another great friend Sue Rowe, principal at Detroit's Christo Rey. I had emailed her about a story I saw on the news about her school. She thanked me for the email and wanted to make sure that I realized that she, as well as the entire student body at Christo Rey, prays for me daily. Once again I am humbled. A couple hundred people whom I have never met and never will, were praying for me because we are all part of God's Family.

June 17th:

"We Beat the Beast" party. Jeannie and I had talked off and on about hosting a party to thank all of the "family" for completing the cancer journey. Tonight's the party. What a joyous occasion. Everyone showed up, if not in person than in spirit! We provided "We Beat the Beast" t-shirts. The shirts were orange, the representative color for kidney cancer. At one point in the evening somebody asked Jeannie where I was. They laughed when she responded, "over there in the orange shirt!" The menu was burgers, dogs, laughter, and fun!! Ryan and Brother Steve manned the grill. Being together was awesome, many tears that night – tears of joy. Anna Fedor, the family photographer, was in the house. She has been with us every step of the way throughout this cancer journey, so it was appropriate for her to be the photographer du jour. She took many awesome pictures. The special picture was of a group shot. She was able to get everyone's face in the shot. Seconds before she snapped the picture, she commanded to the group, everyone reach out and touch somebody. It was a clear demonstration that we were all in this together. Well over 100 people were in attendance for the night that was one of the highlights of the summer. Thanks one and all.

It is always humiliating to be the center of attention. Many people were kind enough to bring gifts, not intended, but certainly appreciated. I want to zoom in and share the words on some of the greeting cards.

Jeannie O'Hara is the family hair dresser and, you guessed it, another GR grad. She, as many folks at her salon, has journeyed through cancer with us. Her card stated, "You are a shining star, there is no limit to what you can do." To which she added, her personal message, "You're amazing." Thanks for the kind words.

My cousins came from St. Clair Shores (where I was born). Their card stated, "Great people accomplish great things." They were excited to celebrate great health. As we get older, we only see our cousins at funeral and weddings. It was so appreciated that they came to join in this special evening.

Anna and Paul are frequent contributors to CB. An old lady was peacefully sitting in her rocker on the front of the card. Inside she is dancing and has thrown off her glasses, while exclaiming, "Hot Damn and Halleluiah." My sentiments exactly. They also brought an applique which I hope to apply to the wall above the bed, whenever I can see straight enough. It says, "Every day holds the possibility of a miracle." Every time I see Sr. Mary Finn, she lovingly looks at me and calls me a miracle. I like that word.

The Kiefer family used their humor when they presented me with a card that says, "It just goes to show ya, almost anything can be fixed with duct tape." They also presented me with a stuffed toy beast that had the words, "I am healed" applied to its midsection in duct tape.

Sue and Vaughn celebrated, "your freedom from cancer and the wonderful gift of friendship. Be patient!" I do not know if there is anyone more blessed than I am with the amazing friends that I have. So many of them/you are always there and their/your support is so needed and appreciated.

Annie Bellino is one of the many nieces and nephews who have walked with me. Her card was phenomenal. She wrote: "What a year it has been. I can hardly imagine the thoughts that have gone through your mind or the conversations you have had with God. Through it all you have been in my prayers! We are all so thankful to have you in the family. This past year, for me, has been a difficult one. I have gained great friendships with the people who've helped me grow stronger in my faith life and I feel truly blessed for that. If I have learned one major thing this year, it's that God has a plan. As much as we want, we cannot allow ourselves to take away the pen from Him as He writes our incredible story. This cancer is now a chapter in your book! Use it to teach others of His works! I have always thought of you as an addictive conversationalist. What you've discovered this past year will only increase that trait ten-fold. May God bless you on this new journey. I love you!" Wow! Thank You, Annie. Thank you everyone. Her words are tremendously inspiring and once again, I am humbled. She closed with the gift of a Bible verse (Jeremiah 29:11-12) which states, "I know the plans I have in mind for you – it is Yahweh who speaks – plans for peace, not disaster, reserving a future full of hope for you." What an awesome verse to share with all of you.

June 18th was the day of our goddaughter's (Mary Catherine) wedding shower. It, too, was held in our backyard, under the same tent. We changed all of the orange flowers to purple. It was quite the elegant affair. Even some men were allowed to brighten up the event. Mary has always been very special to Jeannie and me. It was a true joy to host this event as she prepares for her marriage, a little over a month from now.

On June 24th, I received a special prayer from Kathy. She has become a person in need of all of our prayers as she struggles with cancer. She sent the following uplifting prayer: "God wanted me to tell you, it shall be well with you this coming year. No matter how much your enemies, including cancers, try this year, they will not succeed. You have been destined to make it and you shall surely achieve all your goals this year. For the remainder of 2011, all your agonies will be diverted and victory and prosperity will be incoming in abundance. Today, God has confirmed the end of your sufferings, sorrows, and pain, because He sits on the throne and has remembered you. He has taken away the hardships and given you JOY. He will never let you down." Now let's all pray this one daily.

    It was an honor and a pleasure to be in attendance at the celebration of Fr. Prus's 50th anniversary of priesthood. It was held on June 26th. If you have paid attention, of course you have, you already are aware of what an impact Fr. Prus has played in my life. It was a thrill for Jeannie and me to be invited to his Mass. The church was jammed as many folks have been affected by that spiritual giant. His homily was very effective. He started by walking into the nave of the church and approached the fifth Station of the Cross, his personal favorite. He meditates on it often and I didn't have a clue what it was. Simon of Cyrene helps Jesus carry the cross. We are all called to be Simons. Are we willing to accept? Wow! Great challenge! Fr. Prus then told the story about a young girl who had some challenges in her life. She was able to make him an apron, of which he was quite proud. The apron is the symbol of service, ties right in with the Simon story. With that, Fr. Prus put on the apron and wore it over his vestments during the rest of the Mass. For all I know, he may still be wearing it! What a witness that was. Fr. Prus then told the story of a person whom he was asked to visit in the hospital. He knelt at that person's feet. His comment was that it was an honor to kneel at their feet. What a great gesture – to kneel at their feet. So profound! What a day to spend in honor of a modern day saint. We received an awesome thank you card from Fr. Prus, following his 50th anniversary celebration. His humility is incredible. We wrote words of our adulation in his card. He responded by wondering who we were talking about and he hopes he is able to live up to our words of praise. Of course he can!

    On June 30th I did my normal Thursday routine at Southshore Hospital. I was organizing my paperwork, when the door burst open. As I am always there alone, that was quite startling. Standing before me was Mike Dziuban. Mike has been a long time fellow volunteer; he was returning to service after being off for several months. He is a good guy and it was great to see him. He took one step back and looked at me and said: "What in the world has happened to you?" I was amazed at that comment because I was feeling that life was well on its way back to normal. Was my illness that obvious? I guess so. Mike said I looked weak and he observed the weight loss. I explained to him the details of my cancer journey. Instantly he bowed his head in reverence and we prayed together. The power of prayer is so strengthening. The spontaneity of Mike was so appreciated and genuine. Where would we be without prayer?

Chapter Sixteen
A Month Celebrating Freedom
July

I chose that title for this chapter because it is signifying a return to normalcy. Every day I feel myself getting stronger and winning this war of recovery.

The month started with one of the zanier promotion that Burger King has ever thought up; all of our Original Chicken sandwiches were on sale for $1.04. The logic was that we want to force people into our restaurants. Due to a slumping economy, business has been dismal. The weekend was exciting. It's too early to see the long range results, but hopefully it will have a positive impact. June saw two of the highlights of my Burger King career. Our customers have the option of rating our services through a web-based tool called Guest Trac. In the month of June our final ratings placed us at #2 IN THE NATION for Cleanliness and #9 for drive thru experience. I am so proud of my team, especially since they accomplished this with very little support from me.

On July 9th my sister and her family rode bikes in a local fundraiser for cancer research. It is an event that at least part of their family has raced in for a number of years. This particular year saw them riding as a complete family unit. Patsy opted for the 100 mile route; Bob, Ania, and Jahn opted for the 50 mile route. Had I been present I would have opted for the 5 block route. What made this year's race all the more attractive to me is that they decided to dedicate the race in my honor. Every corner I turn I get humbled by somebody else doing something nice for me. I was there in spirit. Patsy said she "took it easy," whatever that means in a 100 mile race. She said the course took a little over nine hours to complete. What an unselfish attitude on the behalf of the Pio/

White family, and in my honor. Thank You.

On July 14th, Matt, Jeannie, and I toured the campus at U of M Dearborn. We have made quite a few campus visits this summer to help Matt solidify where he would like to go to school next year. Being the cheapo I am, U of M Dearborn ranks first as they are willing to give him a chancellor's scholarship – a full ride for 4 years. Matt has earned that acclaim due to a 4.2 grade point average and a 31 on his ACT – hard work does pay off. Matt is already accepted at that institution as well as at Madonna. He has also toured Albion, Western, and Kalamazoo College. All good choices when he is ready to make up his mind.

July 15 and 16th saw a reunion at Camp Ozanam, the place where romance began for Jeannie and me. The reunion itself was actually on the 16th, but Jeannie and I saw it as a chance for a little getaway, so we went a day early. We visited both Lexington and Port Sanilac and did some reminiscing. We spent three hours at the camp, watching the campers in action. It was great to observe. Although the number of campers is limited due to budgetary concerns, the quality of the care is still outstanding. These kids were having the time of their lives. One never knows what background they come from, but there is definitely a need somewhere and St. Vincent de Paul is happy to step in. The actual reunion was terrific. There were more camp alumni than Vincentians present, reliving lots of old memories. The old staff was even invited on the stage to lead a few songs, including the beloved theme song. Denny Litka was there, a classmate of mine. He was in awe. Those 39 acres hold a special place in his heart. He made the comment to me: "I wanna die here." That kind of came out of left field, but demonstrates how much those hallowed grounds mean to him – it is a symbol of ultimate peace. Another interesting thing happened that day. Mr. Paul Guenther is a former college professor of mine and a current Vincentian. I frequently run into him at Vincentian events. We always have a nice exchange. In college, I was not one of his brighter students. One term I failed my final exam (50% of the grade) and failed the term paper (the other 50%) – how I hated those dreaded term papers. I was trying to figure out how to tell my parents how their son could achieve an F in college, especially since I was a History major. I will never know how Mr. Guenther averaged two Fs to equal a C-, but I will never challenge his math skills. It is always good to see Mr. Guenther. All through college, he was always one of the good guys. He participated in our fraternities and joined our retreats. He truly believed in the mission of Sacred Heart Seminary and did much more than the average lay professor. On the Camp reunion day, Mr. Guenther and Valerie (his wife) were in attendance. They walked behind Rick Klapchar and me as we crossed the bridge that divides Camp Ozanam. Rick and I were discussing my cancer journey and recovery. Later in the day as the Guenthers were preparing to leave, Mr. Guenther approached me and wanted to talk about the cancer journey. He did not know that I had this little side trip. He expressed concern and prayerful support. He then reached out and gave me a big bear hug. Thank you Mr. Guenther, I have appreciated your support for these last 40 years, especially today.

July 21st saw the return of the prodigal son – Joe is home from Vegas for a week. Wow was it ever good to see him and spend time with him. He did not overcrowd his schedule so we spent a lot of quality time with him. He has had a tough year, but has weathered it well. There is light at the end of the tunnel. He has made some great friends in Vegas. He loves his new job, selling advertising -- once a salesman, always a salesman. It is great to have the whole family together. If you don't have family you are lost!

Joe was home for his cousin's (Mary Catherine's) wedding. As you recall we hosted an exquisite shower for Mary a few weeks ago. What a joyous occasion it was; the first of the three Bellino girls to marry. In fact, it is the first cousin on the Bellino side of the family to get married. Perfect is the only word to describe the evening. This diabetic ate more of those wonderful homemade Italian goodies than he should have; they were scrumptious -- so scrumptious that I felt a little extra dose of insulin was in order. I always keep some in the car for just that purpose. Off I went for some needed relief. The Warden was worried as to my well-being – she never stops. She sent Joey to the car to make sure I was ok. I do appreciate the concern, even though it was unnecessary. When we got back to the Hall, the place was buzzing. It seems we missed the highlight of the evening. Joe "Babe" and his daughter performed the most amazing ever daddy-daughter bridal dance. The first part was the typical slow moving, mushy kind of music. Then the DJ broke into "Everybody Dance, now!" and Joe and Mary danced a wonderfully choreographed piece. Everyone raved about it and I was at the car, correcting some errors of bad eating. A great time was had by all. An interesting side light about Mary and Derek's wedding is that their deacon preached about the theme of unconditional love. When we were married 32 years ago, our vows were partially taken from one of John Powell's books all about unconditional love -- a pretty powerful theme and a wonderful similarity.

    The day after those wonderful marital festivities, Jeannie and I attended a retreat day. After years of seminary and IHM retreats, we figured a little mid-course correction would be in line. A major draw for us was that the guest speaker was none other than Sr. Mary Finn, another one of those spiritual giants with whom I have been lucky enough to walk. She was amazing as always. I even appreciated the two times there were breaks for silent prayer. She talked about spending time with homeless folks; she never gives money, but welcomes the opportunity to speak with them, many times in prayer. She talked about how God's first words in Genesis, in dealing with the humans in the universe, center on how good they are. Say this to yourself daily: "And God said ____ (your name) _____ you are very good!" We all need to do that. The other thing that she talked about that impacted me is a new way to say the Hail Mary. In that I frequently pray the rosary, I was all ears. In the last part of the prayer, instead of saying "pray for us sinners," single out the name of someone who needs those prayers. She had two great examples in Tiger Woods and Kwame Kilpatrick. They need our prayers. In praying for them, we shift the focus from thinking/talking about them to praying for them. Let's face it, we all have many names we can insert at that point of the prayer. "Pray for Chuck, your sinner." At the end of the day I felt refreshed.

    In honor of Joe's homecoming, we decided to celebrate on

Sunday, July 24th with a bit of nostalgia. Jeannie, Joe, and I traipsed off to Comerica Park to see Paul McCartney. What a show! Paul performed for three hours on stage without a break – no warm-up act – all Paul. The crowd loved the Old Beatles songs more than the old Wings songs. For the three of us it was also a chance to get together. Joe started the evening with, "we gotta have a talk." Since we have been talking for three days, we didn't know what to expect. Nothing earth shattering, just Joe wanting to share with his mom and dad. He may be 29 years old, but he is still my kid. During the concert I was texting (slowly) with Jay Yule. I asked Jay (whose kids are older than mine): "do we ever stop worrying about our kids?" His quick one word response was "nope"!!

Thought for the day: "Tough times never last, but tough people do!"

Chapter Seventeen

Unfinished Business

When you read a book, do you get tempted to skip ahead to read the ending to see how it turns out? I am guilty. Up until July 16th, there were no surprise endings in store. As I write today I do not know what to expect. On July 16th I received my CT scan results. The test was supposed to be routine to make sure that there were no problems, especially in the kidney area. I passed with flying colors, mostly. Why is there always a "but?" The results indicated two pulmonary nodules on my lungs. One of the nodules is 7mm and the other 8mm. They are very small. When they get to 25mm in size they become dangerous and often cancerous. Dr. Nazareno is not concerned and recommends following up with Dr. Hafez.

I immediately called Dr. Hafez, to be told he is on vacation. I explained the situation to his nurse. She told me that Dr. Hafez is a kidney doctor and could be of no help. She referred me to my family doctor. As the family doc referred me to Dr. Hafez, confusion reigns again. I then explained to the nurse that I would like to keep everything centered at U of M and I asked her to find me a Pulmonologist, so that I could get some action before Dr. Hafez returns from vacation.

This process has dragged out and has been back and forth. The main plus is that nobody is overly concerned about those damned nodules. The nurse at U of M says that the written report refers to them only as, "infectious and inflammable." Sound good to me, but I am still looking for closure.

On July 24th it was decided by the general pulmonology department, that I will have a more detailed CT scan of the thorax (chest) area. We are trying to set that up ASAP, but things never move as fast as one would like. I just got off the phone with Brother T. He was amazed at how calm I am. Do I do a good job faking it? Seriously, I have learned to trust in the Lord. Further, I know that worrying will do absolutely no good. I am better to just keep on pressing forward the time table so we can determine what course of action to take with those two critters.

On July 27th I was assigned a pulmonologist at U of M, Dr. Melissa Kovach. They have set me up for a series of breathing tests on September 2nd. We will have the results of the CT scan long before then. If there is nothing to be concerned about, then we will meet her then. I sure hope that is the scenario.

On July 28th we had another marathon day at U of M. The day started with having my blood drawn. A simple procedure, but it took two jabs; the nurse said the first vein was all dried up. Then we met with Dr. Hafez and his nurse practitioner, Kathleen. They both continued to be amazed by the healing from the cancer surgery. There is no concern about the swelling or numbness – it will take years for that to go away. There were just too many muscles that they had to go through. The nurse said that there is a "binder" that many opt to wear to hold in the swelling. Jeannie laughed and said that women have been wearing them for years and they are called girdles.

At this point I figured the book would end and we would all live happily ever after. Then this scare sprung up about two testy little pulmonary nodules on the lungs. Dr. Hafez said that he thinks this might be "overkill" on his part. While saying that he threw his hands in the air and said, "But, I deal with kidneys and not lungs!" So part one of his statement was well received and part two not so much. I asked him to give me his best estimate on what percentage chance he feels those nodules are cancerous. He would not hazard a guess. He did say that he hopes I am not losing any sleep over this discovery. And I have not. Today did bring about another concern that I have not voiced yet to anyone, except (now) to my readers. When I weighed in I have lost four pounds since May 20th. When you are trying to lose weight that is a good thing, but when you are not trying it gives rise to a scare. I lost 35 pounds in the first three months of the year when cancer was present and then I started putting weight back on.

Now I have lost four pounds. Does that mean cancer is back? Jeannie was amazed because she disapproves of my eating, so do I. We will just have to closely monitor this process. I am scheduled to meet the pulmonologist on September 2nd. Both Dr. Hafez and Kathleen thought that was way too long; they will use their pull to move up that date.

We then discussed the 11th and 12th Commandments. The 11th commandment is: "Thou shalt only have cancer once in a year." And the 12th Commandment states: "Thou shalt only have cancer once in a life time." Two pretty good precepts to live by for me.

We then had a break in the schedule before the chest CT scan. U of M is so large that this one was scheduled at the east Ann Arbor site. It is the third different site we have visited. I loved this place, easy to find and easy to park. We will try to schedule all future testing there. We arrived early so they started early and we were done before the test was scheduled to start. Once again, the nurse has a hard time locating a vein in which to insert the IV. An IV is needed to shoot in a contrasting dye so they can better see the chest cavity. She checked and checked. She walked across the room and removed a heated blanket from the cabinet. She wrapped up my arm in it, to force a vein to pop to the surface – it worked. And then I got to keep that warm blanket for the test. The results will be available on Wednesday and then we have to see if the appointment with Dr. Kovach can be moved up.

Why do kids have to start being responsible at age 29? Joe called at 4:40 AM (Michigan time) to let us know that he had landed safely in Las Vegas. His flight out of Chicago was delayed so he was three hours behind schedule. Glad to know he was OK, but couldn't it have waited?

Saturday, July 30th marked the funeral of Pat O'Grady. I referred to him and his wife, Karla, earlier in this book. I worked for them from 1975-1979. We had lots of fun. Some of the regular CB contributors, (Rick and Sheri Champine and Anne Marie Michels), I met while working there. Pat had some illness problems the last couple of years. The last two days he was breathing with the assistance of a respirator. Once the respirator was removed he went home to Jesus. He is now straightening bar stools in heaven and vacuuming those floors.

The funeral was a great celebration of Pat's life. Pat was the eternal entertainer and a great host – both points were stressed in the eulogy and the homily. Many of the folks I hadn't seen in thirty years; some had gotten older and some, like me, looked even better!

I was given a love tap during the homily. The priest pointed out that today was Fr. Solanus Casey's birthday. It amazes me that, prior to the cancer walk, I had no relationship with Solanus and now I have a deep devotion to the man. I pray for his beatification. The priest pointed out that Solanus had the house job of being the porter, a simple job of service. What a servant he was – wish all of us could resemble those traits.

On August 2nd we received the phone call we were waiting for. Kathleen is the nurse practitioner who works with Dr. Hafez. When we met her last week, we kidded and sparred with each other. But this lady is a professional who really cares and put up with me; we are quite fond of her. She called to say that the nodules that were found recently are "Stable, smaller and resolved" – those are my three new favorite words. She went on to say that there are a few other extremely small nodules, but they are nothing to be fearful of. They are so small that if a doctor wanted to take a sample, it would be impossible as there would be a grave danger that the nodule could be missed and the lung could be punctured instead; that would lead to a deflated lung, which is not a healthy option. Kathleen was going to try and move up my appointment with the pulmonologist, but the report was so positive she does not think that is necessary. WOW! (I recently received a note from one of my "Rocks, Sr. Mary Finn. She explained that WOW stands for "Worthy of Wonder" – pretty special to me.) I have had so many WOW moments and WOW friends; it is a word that I can never wear out.

For a brief time I decided to re-enact Caring Bridge, it is a great way to communicate. I so appreciate the support I have received from so many of my loved ones. Camille said that she was going to light a candle of Thanksgiving to St. Joseph – light the whole candelabra!!

The celebrity doctor, Doctor Oz, tells us that friends are good for our health. Dr. Oz calls them Vitamin F (for friends) and counts the benefits of friends to our well-being. Research shows that people in strong social circles have less risk of depression and terminal strokes. I am so happy that I have a large stock of Vitamin F. Thanks to all of you for being my Vitamin F.

Throughout my life I have felt the presence of God and I have felt the unconditional love of God. God understands me. All I can do is love God, pretty hard to understand him, but Our God is an Awesome God.

My Support Groups

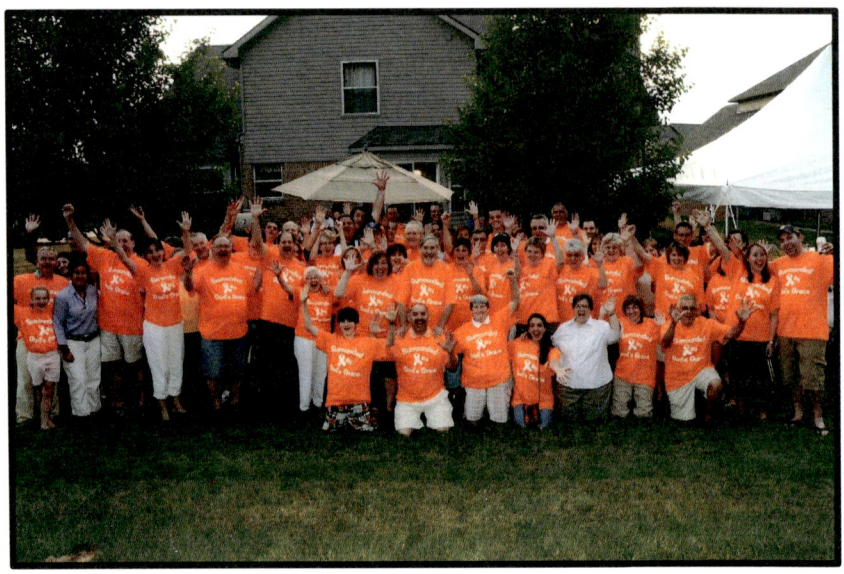

"We Beat the Beast" party
June 2011

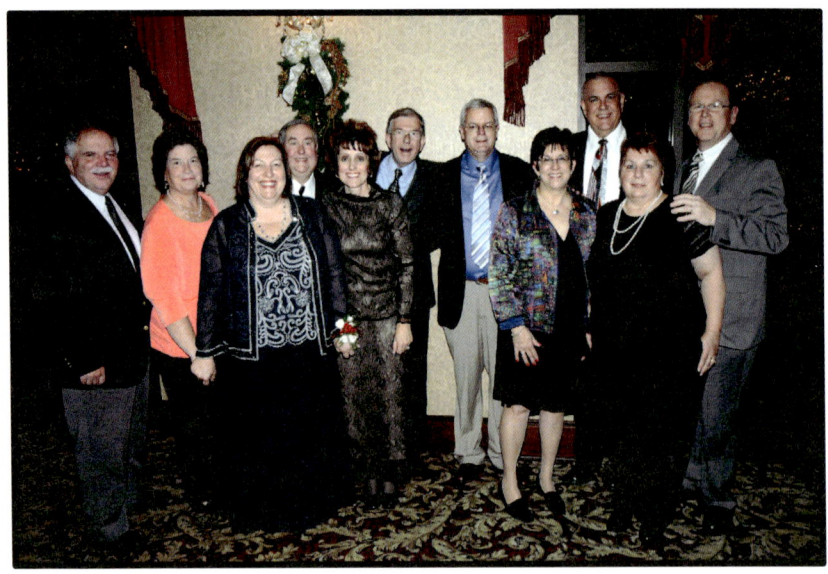

Seminarian buddies and spouses
November 19, 2010

CLOSING COMMENTS

How do you bring a book to its close? Perhaps some of the proof readers who check this out will have ideas.

In the last few days two people have dominated my thinking. The first one is Peg Nichols. She is another camp alumnus who worked with us in the 70's. She recently emailed to announce her 50th birthday and to announce that she had a career change and has two acting parts. The biggest news is that she is cancer free. Five years ago she was diagnosed with advance ovarian cancer and she was given a 20% chance of reaching age 50. Her story is another one of God's love stories. Happy Birthday Peg!

I have decided to refer to the other lady I have been thinking of as "Mary" because I am not sure if she would like her real name to be used. "Mary" is in her mid-30s and is the daughter of great friends of ours. "Mary" has had way more physical challenges than most and is forced to live on disability – she will not be able to work. "Mary" loves life despite her disabilities, and I admire her immensely. Two weeks ago she was raped. Is there any more heinous a crime? What is in God's plans? There are lots of changes coming in "Mary's" life, but she is strong. She is moving to a more secure apartment, which will make all of us rest easier. I have enjoyed communicating with her by email. Although, she has had these challenges, she still loves life and today I received an email picture with "Mary" holding her newest niece, with the warmest smile you can imagine. God is Great! God and the angels were with me and are now with "Mary" and they are with each of you every day!

As I have proofread this book more than once, it serves as a great reminder for me as far as a "to do list." As I get busy, it is very easy to put off important things. I pray for my "family" daily, but sometimes forget to mention some folks individually. So in rereading the entries, I am reminded in the gracious words that you all sent to me collectively and individually. And I am lax with the Gratitude Journal; perhaps, someday, I will make the time to include it more regularly.

Throughout my recovery, I watched too much TV, or should I say I had the TV on too much. This was the 25th and final season of the Oprah Winfrey show. She did have on some phenomenal guests. Other than the Tigers, it was one of the few shows I enjoyed. I figured the final words that Oprah spoke, ending her 25 year career would be an appropriate ending for me as well: "To God be all the Glory!" Amen.

P.S. – Are you allowed to do a Post Script in a book? If you are the author I would think it is OK. Today is February 2nd, 2012. We had an appointment with Dr. Hafez today to go over last week's CT scan results. My heart knew the results would be fine, but the mind gave me a chance to worry. He said the recovery is going smoothly; so smooth that he doesn't want to see me for another year. Originally he had said he would see me every quarter, and now it is only once a year.

"TO GOD BE ALL THE GLORY!"

CONTRIBUTION OPPORTUNITIES

Let's face it we all have a lot of charities ringing our doorbells, sending us letters, calling our phones, etc. And there are only so many discretionary dollars to go around. And we all have our personal favorite charities. I am going to list three options for cancer research donations. I urge you not to take away from Peter to pay Paul. Please do not stop giving to your favorite charities, just to support cancer research. However, if you do have some extra cash, here are three options:

1. Relay for Life – simply go online; many communities have this event in late spring and you can donate to the general event or to a specific walker or even show up and help or walk yourself!

2. The address to donate to University of Michigan is: Office of Development 2800 Plymouth Rd., Building 100 Ann Arbor, MI 48109-2800

3. My sister (Patsy Piotrowski) has been involved for several years with the Prouty organization; their monies support the Norris Cotton Cancer Center in New Hampshire and is connected with Dartmouth. They have a website: info@theprouty.org or you can mail a donation to:

>The Prouty
>1 Medical Center Dr.
>Lebanon, New Hampshire 03756.

You east coasters might want to join in as they have biking, rowing, and walking events. Or you could sponsor my sister.

Please remember – only the **extra** cash!! And God Bless You!!